Older & Wiser

A WORKBOOK FOR COPING WITH AGING

NONIE BIRKEDAHL, M.S.W.

NEW HARBINGER PUBLICATIONS, INC.

Publisher's Note

This publication is designed to provide accurate and authoritative information in regard to the subject matter covered. It is sold with the understanding that the publisher is not engaged in rendering psychological, financial, legal, or other professional services. If expert assistance or counseling is needed, the services of a competent professional should be sought.

Copyright © 1991 by Nonie Birkendahl
New Harbinger Publications, Inc.
5674 Shattuck Avenue
Oakland, CA 94609

Cover design by SHELBY DESIGNS AND ILLUSTRATES
Author photo by David Berry

ISBN: 1-879237-10-5
ISBN: 1-879237-11-3

First Printing December 1991, 6,000 copies

Acknowledgments

The more I write, the more respectful I am of editors. I am most grateful for the editing skills and compassionate support of Nina Sonenberg. I am indebted to Matthew McKay and Patrick Fanning for valuable input into the building of this book, and also to Gayle Zanca for overcoming production obstacles. I want to thank Shelby Tupper for her excellent anatomical drawings. Copy editing is a special skill, and I appreciate the work of Mary McCormick. Thanks also to Gail Perryman for her careful and thoughtful proofreading, and to Otaiwan Day for her meticulous typesetting. There are people at New Harbinger whose names I do not know and whose voices I have never heard, but I know they are there, and I know they contributed in various ways.

My sincere thanks to Joseph Maruca, who made sure my medical facts are correct, to Stephen Axthelm for clarifying diet and cancer issues, and to Marjorie Keely for insights on aging and disability. My appreciation to Horton Hodsen for always being willing to discuss anything, and to Debbie Arcieri for more wisdom than her years would suggest.

And finally, a thanks and a hug for my sister, Joy Currier, who allowed me to discuss her life in detail, and the same for the older-than-me friends and members of my family who have provided me with examples of how to grow older gracefully and with strength.

To my aging yet ageless Danish Prince.

Table of Contents

Introduction

When I was 47 years old, I wanted to learn to cross-country ski. With some difficulty I persuaded my 56-year-old husband to sign up for lessons through the University of Utah. At the first meeting they divided the class so all the younger students went with a vivacious and lovely young teacher who looked to be about 12. Walt and I were the only ones in the second class. Our instructor was a white-haired gentleman of 74. We weren't sure what to expect, but we traveled up the canyon with Mr. Ericson to a parking area where a few other people were strapping on their skis.

We had practiced the cross-country glide on a snow-covered golf course in Salt Lake, and thought we knew what we were about. Mr. Ericson thrust out strongly ahead, while we ploughed behind. Soon Mr. Ericson was half a block ahead of us, effortlessly floating up the slope. At the top he turned around and waited, shaking his head at our laborious progress. As we started up the slope, I immediately fell down. Just as I struggled to my feet, with no help from Mr. E., Walt fell. We finally made it to the top, sugar-coated and panting. We then had a lesson in various maneuvers for climbing, turning, and stopping. I fell seven more times. In this way we traversed the mountain up, down, back, and forth for six hours. When we stopped for lunch, we sat on the roof of a privy, the rest of the building completely buried in snow. Seeing my dismayed look, Mr. E. answered with a gesture toward the forest. I skied, fell, and crawled to the recommended site, dug out a space with my pole, and after falling twice more was able to accomplish my task. Giving up all thoughts of dignity, I abandoned the poles, got down on my hands and knees, and filled in the hole like a puppy burying a bone.

At 4:00 in the afternoon, when we quit for the day, Mr. E. was not breathless, nor was he tired. Walt and I could hardly climb into the car. On the way home he told us that he had been skiing since the age of three, and that he was a cross-country racing coach, and taught winter survival classes. He said he was sure we could learn if we had the proper attitude.

You might think that after a punishing day like that we would give the project up. No way. The glory of being out in the sparkling clean air, smelling the pines, and watching fluffy white clouds idle across a brilliant blue sky was enough motivation for us to continue. We did learn, and it became a favorite recreation for several years until a disability ended it. I still go there in my mind when I want to feel peaceful and calm.

Aging is so individual. Mr. E.'s white hair gave no hint of his youthful vigor. My brown hair and slim figure gave no hint of my ineptitude. In a way I was older than Mr. E.

Aging is not restricted to the last decades of life. You have been aging from the moment you slid gasping into the harsh light of life. Of course you thought nothing of that for years and years. Young people look forward to birthdays with such eagerness and pride. Remember how you wanted to be older each year? At age 20, when I married, I was anxious to become 25 so that I would look more sophisticated. Funny thing is, I don't look sophisticated at 62, but now I don't care to. Do you remember when you began to wish the birthdays would slow down or stop altogether? Do you dread birthdays now? Do you resent changes in appearance and vitality? Are you afraid of what the future will bring?

Such questions as these are what this book is about. This is a practical, task-oriented workbook to help you understand yourself while you are changing in a constantly changing world. You've had good and bad so far in life, and that is the way it will continue — but with a difference. As Mr. E. said to us, I say to you: "You can learn if you have the proper attitude." This is a book about attitudes and about learning new skills. Each birthday does not mean that you lose control of your life. You remain the decision maker, virtually to the last breath. "Ha!" you say, "What about Alzheimer's? What about stroke? What about...?" I say that even in these extreme circumstances you are still making decisions by virtue of having prepared for such unexpected events well in advance. First you need facts. Facts serve you the way proper equipment served us in our skiing lessons.

Facts About Aging

You are one of an elite group. It is predicted that by the year 2030 people over 65 will consitute 20.7 percent of the United States population. Life expectancy will increase well above today's age of 75. That's *average* life expectancy, which means that half the population live beyond 75 right now. Malcolm Cowley wrote a delightful book, *The View From 80*, in which he describes well-known people who have lived productive lives beyond 75. Renoir, who was severely crippled by arthritis, continued to paint with a brush strapped to his arm. Another great artist, Goya, was deaf, and his eyes were so bad that he had to wear several pairs of spectacles, one over another, and used a magnifying glass as well. In spite of these handicaps, he said at age 80, "I am still learning." Cowley believes that, if there were no grave diseases or crippling accidents or inherited defects, the normal life span would be 90 years. Another man who has studied the aging process, Dr. D. D. Stonecypher, offers more good news. He says that even though the body loses 20 to 30 percent of its cells between the ages of 30 and 75, the remaining cells continue to function normally. Did you get that? *Normally.* A 100-year-old person can have a normal electrocardiogram, just like Mr. E's. That's because each red blood cell carries the same amount of oxygen it did when you started out.

Stonecypher discusses some of the physical losses associated with aging and attributes them to loss of reserve, rather than the degenerative process most feared by older people. There are significant differences, just as there were between Mr. E. and me. This means that no two 80-year-olds are alike. My friend Myra, at age 81, drives her car, takes care of her home, and goes swimming three times a week. She is as bright, intelligent, and interesting as my 35-year-old children. On the other hand, Sara, at age 80, lives in a nursing home and can barely walk.

Some of the things you can expect to happen to some degree are these. Your ovaries or testes, as the case may be, will quit manufacturing eggs or sperm. A woman will not likely conceive a child after 70, but I suspect she wouldn't really want to, anyway. Your stomach will manufacture less acid and the lenses of your eyes will become less mobile. That's why you have to get longer arms for reading. You most likely will not have as much tolerance for exercise as you did when you were younger, unless you have been athletic all of your life, like Mr. E.

Your lungs lose some air sacs, your kidneys lose some filtering elements, and your bones get thinner. You won't have as much adrenal hormone, often called the stress hormone, but your body adjusts to these changes. If you stay healthy until 70, your prospects of continued healthy life are good because this process of losing cells, elasticity, and so on, levels off at that age.

Stonecypher declares, "Aging causes almost no disease." Normal old age is healthy, and your mind doesn't have to turn to mush. Your brain can stand a lot of damage without losing intellectual powers — if you have an attitude of optimism, a willingness to keep learning, and you are not afflicted with organic disease.

The health problems that occur in old age are caused by injuries, such as falling off a step stool, or by the same illnesses and infections that happen to people of any age. Improper nutrition can cause disease, and it can impair the body's ability to overcome infections. Some diseases are inherited, and some come about from abusing your body with alcohol, drugs, tobacco, or a failure to exercise. I have systemic lupus. My two aunts in their 80s have it. I have had it since birth, but it did not show up in my aunts until their late 60s. The interesting thing is that there is no difference in the way the disease affects us. Age has nothing to do with our response to disease.

As you get older, you may worry about your memory. Most memory problems are not caused by organic brain damage; they are simply the result of inattention. In fact, many of the problems that can make a person appear to be senile are simply due to stress. The child whose parents have just divorced and who seems to have forgotten how to do sums is no different from the older person whose husband has died and can't remember what bank she uses. Both suffer from stress. You can learn to manage stress. You can learn to change now so that you will avoid future problems. Any problems you do have may be anticipated, and decisions made so that the quality of your life will not be significantly impaired.

The Victory of Age

Florida Scott-Maxwell wrote a book about her 83rd year, *The Measure of My Days*. You might enjoy reading it, as well as others mentioned throughout this book. She experienced infirmities, but still said, "We who are old know that age is more than a disability, it is an intense and varied experience, almost beyond our capacity at times, but something to be carried high. If it is a long defeat, it is also a victory, meaningful for the initiates of the time, if not for those who have come less far." What is she saying? I think she means that you must focus on the moment, be proud of your years, and accept the challenge to be the victor.

You often hear about famous people who have done well into late life. Tolstoy, author of *War and Peace*, lived beyond 80 in an era when life expectancy was around 65. Toscanini, Rubinstein, and more recently Eubie Blake were all performing until their late 80s and 90s. Blake, a ragtime composer, died not long ago at age 100. Rosina Levine, another musician whom I have heard many times at the Aspen Music Festival, was still learning new piano concertos in her later years. I have read that Pablo Casals, the great cellist, had severe arthritis in his 80s, but every morning he hobbled to the piano: slow, bent, shuffling. There he began to play Bach. Gradually his posture straightened; the gnarled hands became mobile so that finally he could take up his cello and make music like no one else in the world.

And what about George Burns? He wrote a book in 1983 called *How to Live to be 100 or More*. He tells about winning a Charleston contest at age 65. When you watch George, you know he is not diminished in the least. He has advice for you: "There's an old saying, 'Life begins at 40.' That's silly...life begins every morning when you wake up."

Ben Franklin helped write the United States Constitution at 81, and Albert Schweitzer was still running a hospital in Africa at 89.

OK, those are famous people. What about older people you know? Some of them may be disabled and some are slow, but I'll bet there are many who are bright, energetic, and as able as someone much younger. Take time now and think about your older friends and relatives. What has happened in their lives to affect the way they live now? What do you want to be like at age 70? 80? 90? 100? This book is written to help you achieve the kind of life you desire as you grow older.

How To Use This Book

I'm fully aware that you will want to shop around in the book, looking for things that are particularly relevant for you, but I want to urge you to read Chapters 1, 2, and 3 first, and to do all the exercises. Everything else in the book depends upon what you do in these three chapters. This is a *work* book. That means the same thing it did when you were in school — except now you're the teacher as well as the student. You'll want to read the material, complete the exercises, and take some time to evaluate your responses. The rewards of an interactive reading will be yours.

Some of the exercises involve filling out a worksheet as you read; some ask you to keep a running worksheet for a series of days or weeks. Don't be afraid to write in this book: that will make it all the more your own personal resource. You might prefer to make copies of the worksheets, or even to take your own blank pages to write on. Some of the exercises just ask you to sit back and reflect. Some — as in Chapters 1 and 9 — involve going to the doctor, or into your community, with new goals. These exercises are important, as you'll realize when you uncover the spirit behind them.

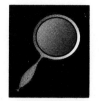 What all the exercises and activities have in common is the opportunity they allow you for concentrated self-reflection. Every time you see this hand mirror symbol, you'll find a self-reflection exercise. The more carefully you look into yourself in completing these exercises, the greater your rewards will be in terms of a new understanding of yourself as a total person in your unique environment. You'll discover how much fun it can be to learn to know yourself more completely and fully than ever before. There is security in knowing.

Now, grab a sharp pencil and some crayons or colored pencils. You are ready to begin Chapter 1.

1

Your Inner Systems

Living Systems

Whenever my father left home, even if it was only to go to work or for an evening meeting, he would say to my mother, "I don't want you to be lonely," and she would say, "Don't worry, I have me, myself, and I." Of course, she also had two children, but I guess father didn't think of us as "company." Mother was right, though, because she knew that even when alone, she did not need to be lonely.

You are much more than just an "I." You are a complex assortment of feelings, thoughts, and behaviors. You are housed in a body that is more intricate than any computer. Even that is not all that you are. You have family and friends, and you live in a designated space in the universe. Something is happening to you, your people, and your space all the time.

This chapter focuses on the intricate innner systems that bring you to life: your physical self. In the next chapter, you'll turn your focus outward, to the network of family, friends, and community that anchor you in the universe. And in later chapters you'll have a look at the mental and emotional processes that connect you to yourself and to the world. All are part of your overall living system.

You might already know how many of your physical systems work — especially if they've caused you trouble. But as you age, it becomes more important than ever to understand the miracle of your body clearly, and *before* trouble strikes. Knowledge brings control. At the end of this chapter, you will be asked to visit your physician, armed with increased knowledge of your own bodily systems. Take this opportunity seriously. Once you have the tools to understand your body better, you can take charge of your physical well-being. You're the one best able to care for your present self and to anticipate your future needs. Remember that you're the true expert on yourself.

When you're happy and well, emotionally all together, life feels good, doesn't it? The problems arise when one of your systems gets out of kilter. Suddenly many systems you hardly thought about prove interrelated, and everything losses its balance. An example will help you see how one push at one level can make that happen.

Margaret's Story

Margaret retired from her nursing job at age 65. Two weeks after leaving her job, she went to a travel agency to pick up brochures about prepaid bus tours for herself and her husband, Harry, to various parts of the United States. Margaret was smiling as she left. Clutching the many papers and booklets, she fumbled to get the car keys out of her purse. Some of the papers fell into the street. Margaret quickly stepped off the curb to retrieve them, and did not see the truck. Horns sounded, brakes squealed, but Margaret knew nothing.

"Your pelvis is broken, Margaret," is the next thing she heard from the kind-looking nurse addressing her in a hospitral bed. "Don't try to move now...you need to rest." Then, seeing the panic in Margaret's eyes, the nurse said, "You're bruised and sore, and I know it's scary, but you must believe me...you are going to be fine."

What will happen to us, Margaret thought. Nothing will ever be the same again.

Margaret was right. Nothing was ever to be the same again. But the nurse was right, too. Margaret's bones healed, and after a long period of treatment and physical therapy, Margaret walked.

Margaret's husband assumed more of the household tasks, which made him a little irritable at times. Margaret felt depressed a good deal of the time, and she began to have thoughts that her husband would be better off without her. Their children's lives were disrupted because they tried to travel home at more frequent intervals. The truck driver, who was not at fault, had a period of suspension from his job, and suffered recurrent dreams of the accident. Margaret saw that an accident to one person upset a lot of other people.

After a time, life assumed a new normalcy — different from the old — but once again balanced and somewhat predictable. Margaret and her family used their experience to train themselves for future unexpected events.

Margaret, like many people, hadn't done much planning for the retirement years. She and Harry were complacent, believing that their pensions and retirement funds would support them adequately. But they had made no preparations for unexpected events.

System Connections

Let's look closely at what happened to Margaret. She thought of herself as primarily being "me, myself, and I," an individual collection of thoughts, feelings, and behaviors. After the accident she began to see herself as part of the larger system, which indeed she was, just as you are and as we all are.

You can see that you are a system, containing many smaller systems, and those systems are populated by even smaller systems such as cells, organelles, and molecules. At the same time, you are part of increasingly larger systems. You have a family, you live in a neighborhood, and you are a part of the world and the universe.

Now, that's not really news. Margaret was certainly aware of it at a deeper level of thinking, but the intimate relationships between the systems had not impressed her until the accident. The important thing to remember about systems is this: when something happens at one system's level, all other systems are affected. In an Indian sand painting, every thin line has significance. To disturb any part of the design would change the meaning of the painting.

When Margaret and Harry retired, that was a change from employment to unemployment. It was an external change that affected the way they lived. Their interests became focused on leisure time. They had to get used to both of them being at home every day. In some ways, their life was carefree. These changes were both external: how their time was filled, where they went each day, and internal: what they thought about, worried about, and planned for.

When Margaret was felled by the truck, her internal systems were directly affected. There was trauma and shock to the brain, nervous system, bones, and muscles. The drugs caused changes in Margaret's biochemistry, and her adrenal glands were stressed by the demand for larger amounts of stress hormone.

Outer systems were also affected. Her husband and children experienced stress and inconvenience. Relationships between the generations shifted to allow the children to assume caretaking roles. Friends and neighbors altered their daily lives in order to help. Harry developed a stomach ulcer.

Insurance carriers felt the impact. Medicare funds were called upon. The entire truck company was impacted by the investigation of the accident. A stepped-up program of stringent driver safety training was instituted. The truck driver suffered emotional trauma and the humiliation of suspension. His family recoiled from the shock.

Beliefs were challenged. Harry had moments of wondering if they were somehow being punished. Margaret, in pain, asked the question, "Why me?" They got into a tiff about who was to blame.

"Why were you so careless?" Harry demanded. "It was foolish to worry about getting those papers out of the gutter."

"I know, Harry, I didn't think," said Margaret.

"That's right, you didn't think, and now look where we are," Harry replied.

A son, overhearing these words, said, "Hold on, you two. Accidents happen. Let's just work on getting things back to normal."

The School Bus Analogy

This theory of living systems has been around for a long time. It all started with a biologist — L.V. Bertalanffy — who observed ecological changes when animal habitats were disturbed. Social scientists stepped in and observed similar patterns in human life and society. Both groups concluded that interrelationships among the components of an organized whole were of fundamental importance in understanding the totality. I call it the "school bus analogy." The inspiration for this idea came from my friend Greta, who drives a school bus.

As I listened to her talk about the responsibilities and vicissitudes of school bus driving, I saw that her situation was a perfect analogy for the relationship of the individual to her living systems. Greta is the driver of her bus. She makes decisions. On her bus are many small people who depend on her for safe arrival. Outside the bus are cars, trucks, bicycles, and pedestrians. All the parents of all the children on the bus are concerned about how the bus functions. Elderly people who are trying to make it across the street care about the bus.

Greta has to be alert, constantly monitoring what the small people inside are up to, what other drivers are doing, where the kid on the bike is going, and dozens of other things. She must pay attention to the sound of her motor, the gas gauge, the speedometer, and messages coming in on the radio.

If the small people act up and get out of their seats, Greta has to pull over and straighten things out. If one of them gets sick and throws up on the floor, that must be attended to. When a small person has accidentally gotten on the wrong bus, a common mistake early in the year, a new decision must be made and a different course of action taken.

Flat tires, ominous noises from the motor, and other mechanical malfunctions may interrupt the journey. When that happens, the small people get restless and upset. The mothers worry and call the school, the bus company, and the police. School officials become nervous, and they call the bus company, too. The bus company has already received word of the problem from other channels, unless the communication system is broken. So they send another bus or a trouble truck.

Life is good when Greta feels well and alert, and when the bus and the small people behave. As long as other drivers mind their driving responsibilities with regard to the bus, life will continue to be good. Greta knows that she can prevent many problems by planning and making decisions in advance. She gets to know the small people and calls them by name. She becomes familiar with their individual behavior patterns, and can sense when one of them is apt to cause trouble. Greta has talked with the parents and the children's teachers. She also keeps the mechanical parts of her bus in good running order. And finally, she has a plan for every possible emergency. She knows just what she will do. She does the best she can every day, and on the weekends she relaxes.

It's time to get to know the mechanics of your own "bus," so you can be the best possible driver. Understanding the workings of your inner systems — the "mechanics" — is the first step; it will free you to focus later on the many other things on your road of life. Your reward will be a stable balance with the world, and a sound state of health.

The Inside Story

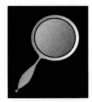 This is a "doing" book, so we're going to start right off with an exercise. Like all the exercises in the book, this is an opportunity for self-reflection, a look in the mirror, if you will. On the following pages are illustrations of the organ systems in your body. Your task is to color each one, any color you want. There are also blank lines for you to describe what you think each organ does. For some, who have studied biology and anatomy, this will be absurdly easy, and you may wonder what such an exercise is doing in an adult book. For others who have less knowledge of anatomy it will seem difficult. Don't either one of you give up and toss the book aside. This exercise is not intended to teach a textbook picture of your insides. It is an emotional experience to help you get in touch with how you, as an individual, perceive the functioning of your body. In the past, I have taught medical students who had a hard time with this because they were bent on getting everything the exact color it is in textbooks and cadavers. Believe me, the colors in a cadaver have small resemblance to the colors in a living body. The *right* colors are those which spontaneously pop into your mind. Those are the colors that will have meaning for you.

It's a good idea to begin with the coloring part of the exercise. The act of taking crayon in hand and physically applying the color to the picture turns the key in your brain that lets you *know*, with your nerves, your muscles, and your emotions, what your body is doing. It makes it possible for you to evaluate whether something inside is getting sick, or just needs a rest.

Try not to process everything. Don't spend time thinking about what color things are. Just sit down with the book, pick up a crayon, and color. Set all reason aside. Pretend you are five years old, coloring for the pure joy of coloring. Your deeper mind knows what it's doing, and it doesn't need any interference from your intellect.

Once you've finished coloring, jot down your thoughts on the different organ systems under the "function" headings. You don't need to be overly specific or formal — just write enough for you to know how far your knowledge extends into each system. I predict you'll have a good time.

BRAIN & NERVOUS SYSTEM

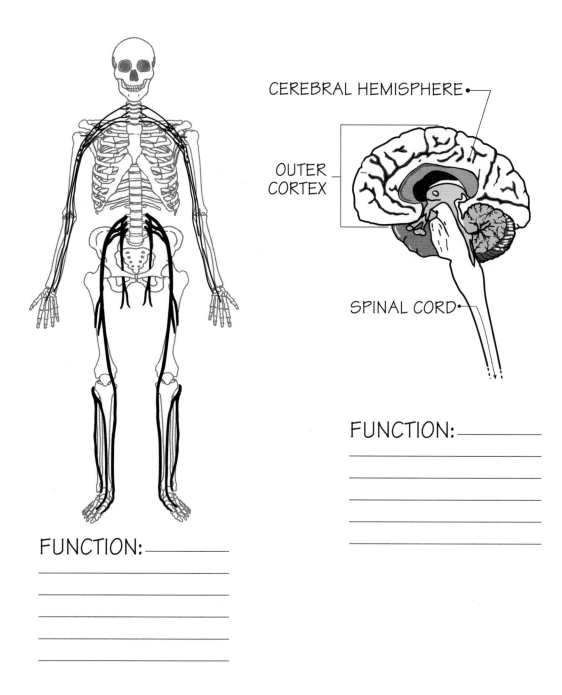

CEREBRAL HEMISPHERE

OUTER CORTEX

SPINAL CORD

FUNCTION: ———
————————————
————————————
————————————
————————————
————————————

FUNCTION: ———
————————————
————————————
————————————
————————————

HEART
[CARDIOVASCULAR SYSTEM]

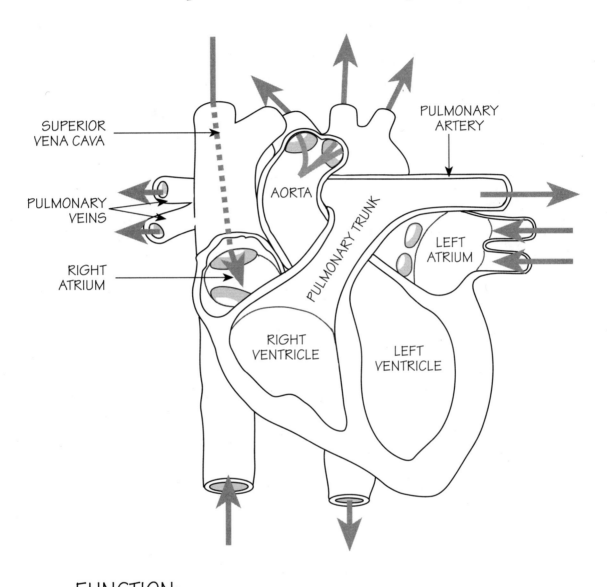

SUPERIOR
VENA CAVA

PULMONARY
VEINS

RIGHT
ATRIUM

AORTA

PULMONARY TRUNK

RIGHT
VENTRICLE

PULMONARY
ARTERY

LEFT
ATRIUM

LEFT
VENTRICLE

FUNCTION: _____

_____

_____

_____

CIRCULATORY SYSTEM
[CARDIOVASCULAR SYSTEM]

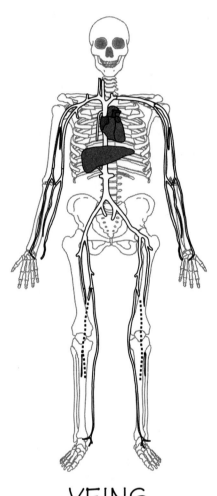

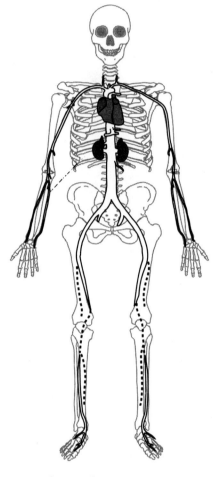

VEINS

ARTERIES

FUNCTION: ————
————————————
————————————
————————————

FUNCTION: ————
————————————
————————————
————————————

RESPIRATORY SYSTEM

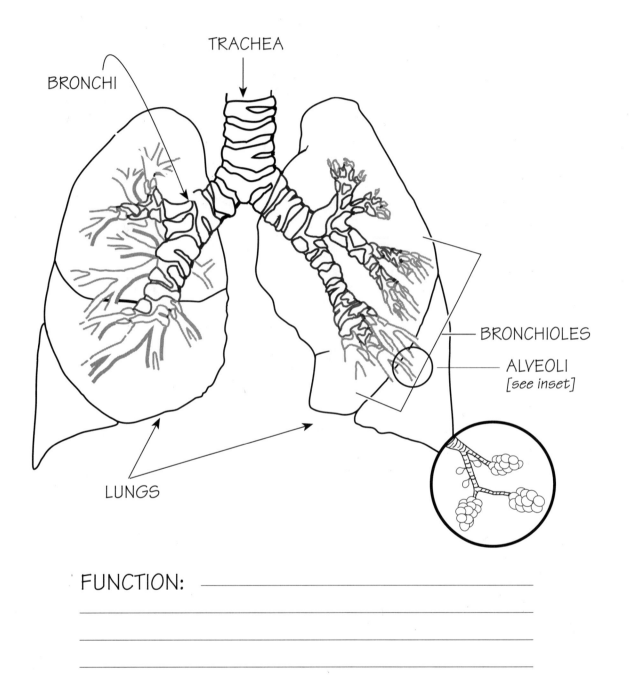

TRACHEA

BRONCHI

BRONCHIOLES

ALVEOLI
[see inset]

LUNGS

FUNCTION: _____
_____
_____
_____

DIGESTIVE SYSTEM

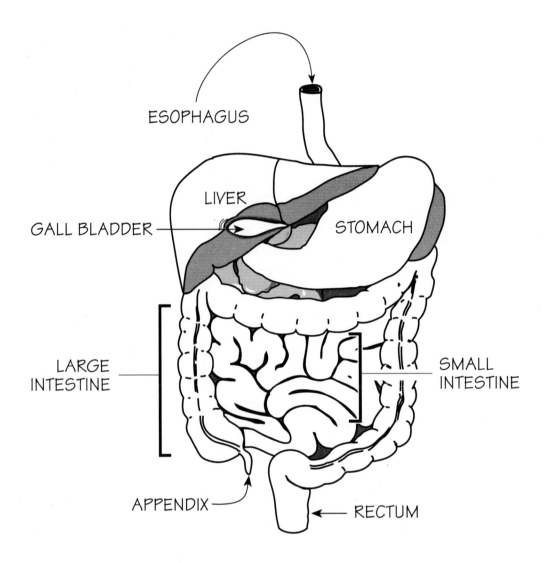

ESOPHAGUS

LIVER

GALL BLADDER

STOMACH

LARGE
INTESTINE

SMALL
INTESTINE

APPENDIX

RECTUM

FUNCTION: _____

_____

_____

_____

BLADDER & KIDNEYS

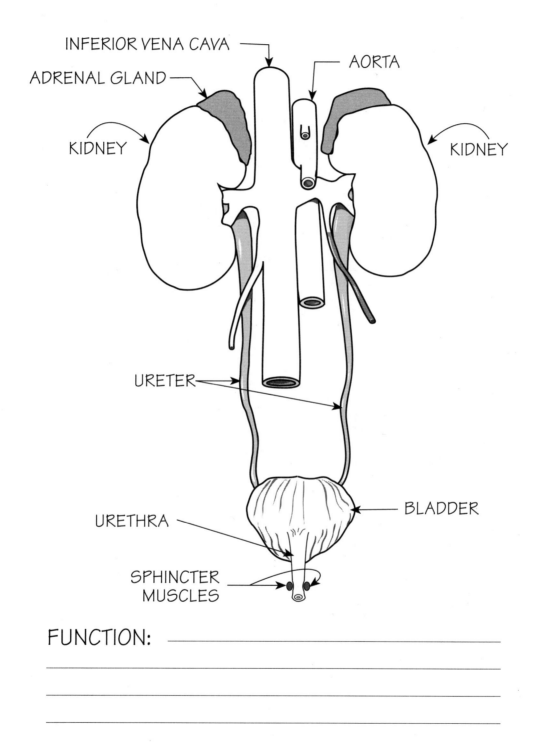

INFERIOR VENA CAVA

ADRENAL GLAND

AORTA

KIDNEY

KIDNEY

URETER

BLADDER

URETHRA

SPHINCTER
MUSCLES

FUNCTION: _____

_____

_____

_____

ENDOCRINE SYSTEM

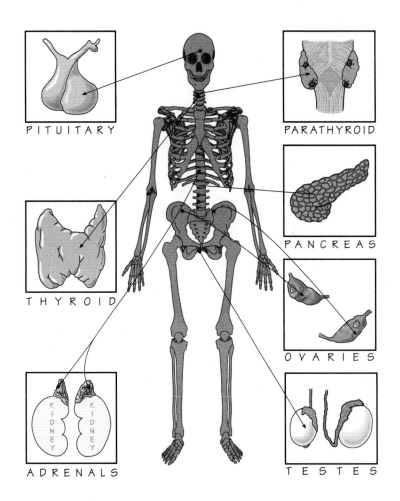

PITUITARY

PARATHYROID

PANCREAS

THYROID

OVARIES

ADRENALS

TESTES

FUNCTION:

PITUITARY: _____

THYROID: _____

ADRENALS: _____

PARATHYROID: _____

PANCREAS: _____

OVARIES: _____

TESTES: _____

MUSCULOSKELETAL SYSTEM

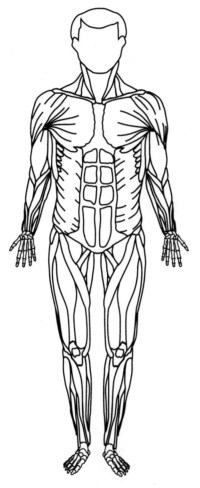

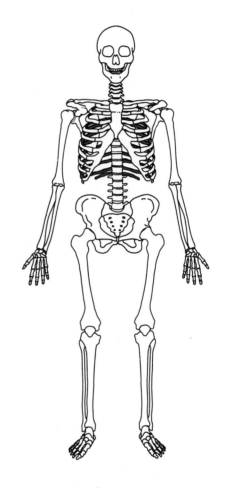

MUSCLES

BONES

FUNCTION: —————

————————————————

————————————————

————————————————

————————————————

FUNCTION: —————

————————————————

————————————————

————————————————

————————————————

IMMUNE SYSTEM

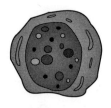

MACROPHAGE

FUNCTION: _____

_____

_____

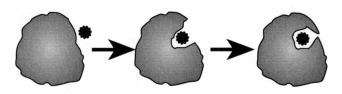

PHAGOCYTES

FUNCTION: _____

_____

_____

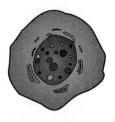

LYMPHOCYTES
[T-LYMPHOCYTES]

PLASMA CELL
[B-LYMPHOCYTES]

FUNCTION: _____

_____

_____

FUNCTION: _____

_____

_____

What colors do you see in your drawings? You might think about what you colored darker, and what you made bright. Did you skip any systems or organs entirely? If so, it might be a sign that you should take a closer look at that system's function and health. Look over your drawings now, and see what you can read in them.

One woman, Caroline, colored her brain bright orange, and her blood cells deep purple. Her kidneys were green, and her heart was blue. Think about a blue heart. Caroline was depressed, but she also had poor circulation. She didn't know that…she just knew that was the way she pictured it. When Caroline's daughter colored her own heart, it was brown. Everyone has different, emotionally dictated colors for the parts of their body. I have blue eyes, but in certain moods I think of them as brown. You don't need any reasons for the color of your heart, or your kidneys, or your ovaries. This was purely an emotional response. Just remember to keep your emotional insights in mind as you consider the actual functions of the systems.

Look over your function notes now. Do you now have an idea about how much you actually know and what you need to learn? Brief descriptions will follow, but your interest may be piqued enough to want more. Some sources for further reading are listed in the references section at the end of the chapter. Public and college libraries can supply you with just about anything you need. Hospitals have libraries, too, and nowadays they welcome visitors. This has not always been so. I remember an incident that happened 25 years ago when I went into a medical library hoping to look something up. The woman there said, with great reluctance, "Well, I'll help you find it as long as it doesn't have anything to do with your own medical problems." How bizarre. Fortunately, these archaic attitudes have changed, and the medical profession not only accepts but also encourages self-education on the part of the patient. You need not be timid about going into a medical library.

For the most part, the following discussion repeats the order of the illustrations. It's the same order you'll find on the physician's report at the chapter's end: from the larger vital systems to the supporting systems. A few things are different below. Some systems such as the lymphatic are discussed but are too small to illustrate clearly. Another important system, the reproductive, is discussed in combination with other systems (ovaries and testes are glands, and so go in the endocrine system). One more difference: I prefer to discuss the most important system — the brain and nervous system — last. I think you'll see why.

Although the discussion addresses each system separately, never lose sight of the fact that all systems work together. What goes wrong in one system affects every other system. Remember the school bus.

Cardiovascular System

Your **heart** has four chambers, as you saw on your heart illustration. Two chambers are called ventricles, right and left, and the other two are right and left atria. The atria accept blood to the heart and transfer it to the more powerful ventricles. The right atrium accepts blood from the great veins (not pictured; they'd be in the upper left) and transfers it to the right ventricle. The right ventricle pumps blood to the lungs, where it can release carbon dioxide and collect oxygen. Blood returns from the lungs to the left atrium and is pumped throughout the body by the powerful left ventricle. **Veins** always carry blood to the heart; **arteries** take it away. The primary veins are called the **inferior vena cava** (receiving blood from the lower half of the body) and the **superior vena cava** (receiving blood from the upper half of the body). The **aorta** is the primary artery.

As the **blood** makes its journey, delivering oxygen and nutrients, it picks up carbon dioxide and other waste products, taking them to the liver and kidneys to be disposed. The blood also carries hormones so that every part of the body can communicate with other parts. The illustration of the circulatory system gives you an idea just how your blood travels within your body. As you can see, it is impossible to talk about one system without referring to others. If you get sick from something wrong with your heart, you are not just "the cardiac case in room 2." You are a complete *person* who is ill.

My sister has a faulty heart. Her heart is paced wholly by a mechanical pacemaker. Recently, after nine years, her pacemaker failed, and she fell over. You can't remain standing if your pump isn't working. She was taken to the hospital, where a new pacemaker was installed. The surgeon, who never saw her before, or after, said to her while she lay waiting, "It's a mechanical procedure. I'm just the mechanic." He acted like a mechanic, too. His only interest was in getting the technology to work. Fortunately, she also has a compassionate and caring cardiologist, who recognized the effect of this trauma on the rest of her system and on her family. It turned out well. She is livelier and better than ever. We needed the mechanic, but we also needed the caring doctor.

Basically, there are three kinds of blood cells: white, red, and platelets. (Or green, purple, and orange if that's the way you see them.) Red cells carry oxygen, white cells fight off disease, and platelets make blood clots. You will learn more about how these cells function under the description of the immune system later in this chapter.

Respiratory System

Lung tissue is very different from heart muscle. The **lungs** do not work on their own the way the heart muscle does. When you take air into your windpipe, it travels through a series of smaller and smaller pipes until it reaches tiny air sacs which feather out inside the lungs. These sacs are called **alveoli**. Each one is surrounded by a filigree of blood vessels — this is where carbon dioxide passes out of the blood, and oxygen is absorbed into it. The soft spongy lungs are protected by the rib cage (not shown on illustration). Muscles between the ribs contract when you want to take a deep breath.

Breathing out is easier than breathing in. When breathing out, all the muscles relax and the lungs contract on their own because of the elastic tissue around them. Notice on the respiratory system illustration that the alveoli are in the deeper parts of the lung, away from the midline. You can see why it is important to breathe deeply so that every little air sac can be filled for the important oxygen and carbon dioxide exchange. If you only breathe shallowly, many alveoli remain collapsed, resulting in poor gas exchange and promoting pneumonia. This situation is most common after surgery or with sedatives and pain medications. It can also occur when you are frightened and anxious. Your posture has a good deal to do with inefficient breathing, too. Mother knew what she was talking about when she told you to "stand up straight."

Claudia, a police dispatcher, actually experienced atelectasis — collapsed alveoli — as a result of shallow breathing. Her job was highly stressful and her energy reserves had diminished over the years. She had become increasingly tense and anxious about her ability to meet the demands of her job. She did not realize that the anxiety was causing her to breathe shallowly. It didn't take long to get back to normal after she learned how to breathe correctly.

Lymphatic System (not pictured)

In addition to the blood circulating system, the lymphatic system also has a circulating network. Lymph is a watery fluid that surrounds and feeds the cells. It fills the spaces between groups of tissues and is made of water, white cells from the blood, and nutrients. Lymph doesn't have a pump, and can only circulate as your muscles contract. If you have ever had swollen feet from sitting on an airplane too long, you have experienced a pooling of lymph. In other words, the muscles in your legs haven't been working, so the lymph can't circulate. Lymph nodes, or glands, are usually very small, about the size of a pea. (That's why they're not pictured.) Their job is to remove germs that have been collected by the circulating lymph. They also make lymphocytes, the cells that fight infection, and antibodies, proteins produced in the body in response to antigens. If there is a problem with your lymphatic system, your doctor will record it under either the immune system or the endocrine system on the chart at this chapter's end.

Long, long ago, when most of us were children, virtually no one made it to adulthood with **tonsils**. It was almost routine to snatch out the child's tonsils if they looked large or unduly red. The function of the tonsil was not well understood. Nowadays tonsils are only removed if they become infected too often or remain swollen too long. Tonsils are cleverly located at the back of the throat to trap germs. The reason they swell is because they are busy getting rid of little invaders. Fortunately, if they do have to be removed, other lymph glands are able to do their work. Most doctors now feel it is better to leave them alone, if possible.

Digestive System

Digestion begins as you break down food by chewing it, and mixing in saliva. Saliva contains enzymes, which initiate the chemical changes necessary for the absorption of nutritional substances. After you swallow, the food passes down the **esophagus** into the **stomach**. There, stomach muscles contract to churn acid juices into the food. As the food becomes liquid, it passes into the **intestinal tract**. Fruit leaves the stomach in about 30 minutes; vegetables take a little longer; and it takes two or three hours to digest meat enough to leave the stomach.

The food, which now bears no resemblance to what you put into your mouth, is further broken down in the **small intestines**. Water and nutritional substances are absorbed into the bloodstream and distributed to all parts of the body. Whatever is left over that the body can't use passes into the **large intestine** and out of the body through the **rectum**. What you eat is so important. If you eat junk, that's what your cells will get.

Here again lies an often removed organ, the **appendix**. In the past, it was thought to be a remnant from some previous period in man's development, but now scientists recognize that it serves a purpose similar to that of the tonsil, although it is not a lymph node. If your appendix becomes red and inflamed, resulting in fever and changes in the white blood cell count, it will usually have to be removed.

Don complained of pain in his stomach. He had convinced himself that he had stomach cancer. X-ray studies were negative, but still Don had this burning in his stomach. "I'll tell you what," said Don's doctor, handing him a diagram similar to the picture of the digestive system which you colored earlier, "take a look at this picture and point to where the pain is." Don pointed to the lower end of the esophagus.

"It's right there, doc," he said. "That's exactly where it is."

"Well, well. That's not your stomach, is it?" asked the doctor.

Then the doctor had Don lie down again and pressed where Don had pointed on the picture.

"This is where your esophagus is, Don, and this," pressing a little lower, "is your stomach."

"Oh. Does that mean I have cancer of the esophagus?" asked Don.

The doctor chuckled. "It's not likely. Let's treat it for two weeks as if it were esophagitis, an inflammation, and hold off on the tests."

That sounded good to Don, who hated any kind of medical procedure. Medication was prescribed along with a diet and some advice about stress. Two weeks later Don came back.

"No pain now," he said, "I feel a hundred times better. Boy, was I scared."

One of the reasons to better understand your anatomy is so that you don't scare yourself to death whenever you feel pain. When you do consult a doctor, you can be more specific about what you are experiencing, particularly after you learn to listen to what different parts of your body tell you.

The **liver** is a large organ that doesn't pump, doesn't have muscles, and doesn't look like much; it just lies there under your ribs on the right side. Nevertheless, it is an amazingly efficient organ that carries out more than 500 tasks. Everything you put into your mouth is processed by the liver. If there is something toxic in your food, the liver will render it harmless. It changes some of the chemicals the body has made from food so they can be used quickly. The liver stores some of these things for future use. Old red blood cells are processed by the liver, and iron is removed so that new cells can be made.

The liver also makes bile, which changes fatty, greasy food into useful nourishment. The bile is stored in the **gall bladder** and drips into the intestine. The liver can be overwhelmed if you give it too much of something potentially toxic. That's why alcoholics get cirrhosis of the liver. Alcohol is a toxin, a poison to the body. Paradoxically, that is also how drugs work. If you have arthritis, aspirin may be prescribed in doses so large that the drug can't be detoxified. This allows the drug to suppress certain chemicals in your body, thereby relieving inflammation and pain. It's good to be aware of this so that you give some thought to what kinds of things you want to put into your body. It does not mean that prescribed drugs should never be used; it means they should be used with caution. Drugs are often necessary and beneficial, but they are not harmless. They can also overwhelm the kidneys' filtering system. It's up to you to be informed about drugs, and to discuss the benefits and side effects with your doctor.

There is one more organ that is considered to be a part of the digestive system, the **spleen** (not pictured). It has other functions, such as producing white blood cells to fight disease, storing blood that can be released quickly when you need it, and making antibodies. It is just a small organ behind the stomach and close to the liver. Like the liver, it breaks down old red blood cells.

Bladder and Kidneys

Sixty percent of body weight is water. Half of that lies inside the cells. The rest is mixed with salt, and bathes the cells. This surrounding fluid must be maintained in a delicate balance. If you place a drop of blood in tap water, the water will rush into the cells, and they will burst. On the other hand, if the blood is placed in a 5 percent salt solution, the salt will pull water out of the cells, causing them to shrink. If either of these changes were to occur inside your body, you could die.

Nearly all cells are surrounded by a network of capillaries from which blood plasma passes into the surrounding fluid by diffusion. One writer calls this fluid the "internal sea." This salty fluid carries nutrients to the cells and removes waste products, which diffuse back through the capillary walls to mix with other blood constituents. When proteins are broken down to provide energy, ammonia is formed as a waste product. Ammonia is a poisonous gas that dissolves in water — one thousandth of a milligram per liter of blood is sufficient to kill you — so it must be eliminated as fast as possible. First the liver converts the ammonia into urea and then sends it along to the kidneys. Urea is also a poison, but the body can handle more urea than it can ammonia. Eliminating urea and balancing the salt in the internal sea is the job of the **kidneys**. They process and filter fluids, producing urine which contains unwanted substances. Urine is eliminated by the **bladder**. Survival of the whole body depends upon the delicate balancing act performed by the kidneys.

The urine drips down the **ureters** into the bladder, where it is stored until discharged through the **urethra**. The bladder, under normal conditions, is capable of holding 700 to 800 cc of urine. Usually, when about 400 cc has collected, a message is sent to the central nervous system, which tells the *internal* sphincter to relax. At that point you get the message loud and clear that you need to empty your bladder. You have conscious control over the *external* sphincter, and it usually will not relax unless you tell it to. Relaxation of the external sphincter allows the urine to pass out of the body by way of the urethra.

If the muscle is weak, you might not be able to control the sphincter. Many women have some problems with leaking after childbirth, and both men and women may have poor control in later years. There are solutions to this problem. You can wear the big people's diapers June Allyson advertises on TV, for one thing. You can also do the Kegel exercise to strengthen the muscle. This exercise consists of tightening all of the muscles around the urethra, vagina, and anus, and then relaxing. Do it this way: tighten, hold 3 counts, relax, and repeat 5 times. Do this 4 times a day. This exercise has helped many people improve bladder control.

Certain kinds of stress may have just the opposite effect — you might not be able to relax the external sphincter, a situation destined to create anxiety and great discomfort. Surgical procedures can do it, anesthetic agents can do it, and emotional distress can do it. The bladder can be stretched to hold 1,500 cc, but that is extremely painful. I have to tell you a sequel to the story of my cross-country skiing experience.

A Painful Lesson

In May, when the ski season was over, I decided to go on a desert survival trip. This was a bad decision. We were allowed to take one wool blanket, a canteen, and just a few packets of dried food. We drove down to southern Utah and began our hike. We walked miles across the sand and slick rocks. It was hot. Little sips of water were not all that helpful. We forded a river two or three times, which was cooling, but then the water squished into our boots and sand stuck to our skin. We rappelled off a cliff, a first-time experience for me, and forded another river. We then followed the river up a canyon. It was tough going, and it was a long day for people who normally spend their days walking around hospitals or sitting in offices talking to people. Finally, we got to a place to spend the night. We brewed up a sort of stew over a campfire, washed in the river, and went to bed. Bed was a hollowed out place in the sand where we could wrap up in our blankets. The air turned cold very quickly. As the night wore on, I became sleeplessly aware that I had a problem other than the 19 million tiny rocks in my bed. I kept getting up to empty my bladder, but nothing happened. I grew increasingly more uncomfortable.

By morning I was anxious. One of our group was a nurse at the same hospital where I worked. I approached him and said quietly, "I have a problem."

"What's that?" he said, eyeing the campfire, where he would clearly have preferred to be.

"I haven't been able to void all night and I'm very uncomfortable," I replied.

"Oh my, we'll have to make you some Brigham tea," he said. (Brigham tea is made from a plant that grows all over the place down there.)

By the time the tea was made, others in the group were aware of my plight, much to my embarrassment. Everyone watched with interest as I drank the tea. Then we all waited expectantly. I drank more tea.

"Drink a lot of tea," they urged. "Just keep drinking."

So I drank more tea. My bladder was getting fuller and fuller, and I waddled as I walked.

A conference was held about whether or not to abort the rest of the trip. Against my wishes it was agreed that if one had to go back, all would go. So we started the long trek back. I made frequent sorties into the brush and behind rocks, but nothing happened. There is no way to describe what it felt like to hike down that canyon and wade through the rivers with such a full bladder. One of my fellows was disgusted and said, "All women have these problems; she'll be all right."

Eventually we came to the cliff we had previously rapelled. They all looked at me and shook their heads.

"There's another way out," said one. "We can climb this sand hill."

I nodded, and we began. The sand was deep. Every step set the sand to sliding so that we slid back more than we went forward. The younger people who had stronger legs were able to make fairly steady progress. I not only was older and less strong, but I also had this huge watermelon in my belly. I did find out, however, that if I took a step and stood perfectly still, I would not slide. So that's the way I made it up that long hill. Step...wait...step...wait. Then we made the long walk back over the flat rocks to the trucks.

The nightmare ended in the emergency room of a small town, where 1,300 cc were drained from my bladder. I felt great, but my friend, who was waiting for me, said I looked a lot thinner. It took a couple of weeks to get back to normal. It was a good experience in a way, because I learned something about how my body reacts under physical duress.

Endocrine System

You have had plenty of experience with hormones. Sometimes you've thought you had too many, sometimes too little. For teens and women, the great cop-out for bad behavior has been, "It's hormones!" And sometimes it is.

The endocrine system is made up of **glands**. Glands are groups of specialized cells that make chemicals for growth, reproduction, and many other essential functions. Some hormones produce short-term, day-to-day, or hour-to-hour changes, while others have long-term effects.

Some glands produce obvious changes in the body — for example, the development of breasts, or mammary glands. Although not formally a part of the endocrine system, you have secretory glands that make you sweat on a hot day. You produce tears in your eyes, not only for crying, but for keeping them moist. That's something that may diminish as you grow older. You have saliva to moisten your mouth and for digestion. Saliva also helps fight tooth decay.

The **pituitary**, which is actually an exocrine gland, hangs down from the base of the brain. It functions under the direction of the hypothalamus, which is described below. It is tiny but mighty because its chemicals act as triggers for other glands to work. The pituitary controls salt concentrations in the blood and helps control blood pressure. It tells the infant's body how fast to grow and when to stop. It determines when a baby will be born. It is a most interesting gland, miraculous when it works correctly, and devastating when it does not.

Chang, a Chinese giant who lived in the 1800s, is one famous case of the pituitary putting out too much growth hormone. He grew to twice the height of his fellows.

My friend Agnes had a strange thing happen to her around her fiftieth birthday. All of a sudden her hands and feet began to grow. She was a petite lady, but her hands became man-size, and her feet grew from size 6 to size 9. She didn't like it. In fact, she became self-conscious about her appearance, and refused to go out for a while. She thought people would think she was a side-show freak. The truth was that very few people even noticed. Of course they noticed when she pointed it out to them, as she was quick to do. She thought if she mentioned it first that people would be more accepting. She received some medical treatment, and after a while she got over her self-consciousness and could go out and enjoy her friends. She still had big hands and feet, but no one cared.

The **hypothalamus** (not pictured), located inside the brain above the pituitary, actually controls the thyroid, adrenals, and gonads glands, plus lactation and growth. It does so through the pituitary, which is actually only a transmitter of hypothalamus control. The hypothalamus also controls biologic rhythms, such as sleep and wake cycles, menstrual cycle, timing of puberty and growth spurts, appetite, metabolism, temperature, and hydration.

At the bottom of the throat lie the **thyroid** and **parathyroid** glands. Everyone knows about thyroid. There was a time, and I'm sure you remember it, when thyroid supplement was given for weight control. The theory was that it would speed up metabolism and burn more calories with less effort. The kicker in this plan was that by giving extra thyroid, the gland more or less said to itself, "Hey, I don't need to do anything. I'll just quit working." By the time this was realized, a lot of people had inefficient thyroid glands. The thyroid has a good deal to do with the amount of energy you have, and if you get too much thyroid, you will become restless and overactive. During pregnancy, you probably took iodine or some iodine-containing supplement. That was because the developing fetus does not make any thyroid of its own until about 12 weeks. Lack of thyroid in the fetus results in a state of mental retardation known as cretinism.

The parathyroid provides a hormone for muscle strength and for bone and calcium metabolism. Calcium is essential for teeth and bones. Most of the calcium in your body is in your bones, but some is circulating in the blood. Calcium is essential for many vital functions. Therefore, calcium can be drawn out of the bones when needed elsewhere. A hormone known as parathormone increases this movement of calcium from bone to blood, the amount dependent upon the need. Circulating calcium plays a role in blood clotting, contraction of muscles, and the action of nerves. Deficiency of calcium makes the muscles contract uncontrollably, resulting in a potentially fatal condition called tetany. Calcitonin, a hormone secreted by the thyroid, does the opposite. It encourages the movement of calcium from the blood into the bones. Sometimes people with osteoporosis are given calcitonin for this purpose.

Adrenal glands are so-called because "renal" refers to kidney, and "ad" means next to. These glands sit on top of the kidneys like caps. The most essential function of the adrenal is to produce cortisol. Without cortisol you would die in 72 hours, although its exact function is a mystery. The adrenals also produce aldosterone, which controls salt conservation. From the inner layer of the glands, other hormones, the catecholamines, are produced in response to pain, fear, and other emotional disturbances, as well as when increased muscular effort is needed.

Think about the last time your phone rang at 2:00 a.m. What was your first thought? Something wrong with one of the children? Is it the hospital calling about your seriously ill brother? You probably awakened pretty quickly because you had an increased amount of adrenal hormones pouring into your bloodstream.

The crises you are most apt to face do not call for physical effort. The actions you will have to take are mental, but your adrenals pour out enough adrenaline to help you fight a mountain lion — both physically and mentally.

Other hormones are secreted by the adrenal cortex. Glucocorticoids are secreted in response to a hormone released by the pituitary, ACTH (adrenocorticoid hormone). The one most people are familiar with is hydrocortisone, which regulates carbohydrate, protein, and fat metabolism. It also has a powerful anti-inflammatory effect. This hormone is routinely given when there is head injury because it reduces swelling in the brain. If you have rheumatoid arthritis, systemic lupus, or another autoimmune disease, you may have been given prednisone, a synthetic form of hydrocortisone. Back in the 1940s, this drug was heralded as a miracle drug because it so dramatically reduced the pain, swelling, and stiffness that go with these diseases. When the side effects appeared, they were serious. Prednisone suppresses normal adrenal activity. Consequently, you can't stop taking it suddenly because your own adrenals won't be functioning as they should. You could have adrenal insufficiency and become seriously ill. You could even die if not treated promptly. This drug robs your bones of calcium, creating osteoporosis — the fragile bone disease. It also changes your appearance, giving you a moon face and unwanted deposits of fat on your body.

Other adrenal hormones regulate sodium levels and volume of fluid. Gonadocorticoids are sex hormones, one of which is androgen, an important hormone in women for regulating libido and aggression.

Ovaries and **testes** function in a way that is well known: they provide sex hormones. As an older woman, your ability to produce viable eggs and conceive a child is waning, or gone. If you are a man, you still produce sperm beyond the age of 70, but the sperm become increasingly less mobile, and fewer in number. These events do not affect sex drive, however. Sexual function in the male depends upon vascular and neurologic factors in addition to hormones and libido. Erectile impotence caused by vascular or neurologic factors can be corrected or facilitated with nonsurgical or surgical solutions. On the Living Systems Inventory, *Inner Systems*, at the end of this chapter, your doctor will indicate the health of these glands under the reproductive system heading.

Have you seen the Kathryn Hepburn movie, *Mrs. Delafield Wants to Marry*? Hepburn plays the part of an aging woman, a widow who falls in love with an equally aging man. Much against the wishes of her family, Mrs. Delafield decides to marry. Religious conflict enters in, which upsets both families even further. But the most shocking thing for Mrs.

Delafield's children is learning that this aging, wrinkled mother feels passion and sexual desire when her husband-to-be kisses her. Sagging flesh and white hair are not indicators of sexual ability.

The **pancreas** is the gland that secretes insulin, essential for decreasing blood sugar. It also decreases blood potassium and phosphate levels. Glucagon, on the other hand, is a hormone secreted to increase blood sugar, convert proteins and fats to glucose, and increase blood potassium and phosphate levels. The right amount of each is necessary to maintain balance.

Basically, the system works like this: when the blood sugar rises to a certain level, insulin is secreted to keep it from going any higher. When it works, it works very well, but, like the little girl with a curl in the middle of her forehead, when it's bad, it's horrid. When insulin is not secreted, or when the body cannot properly use insulin, the person is said to have diabetes.

Diabetes

Type I diabetes usually begins in childhood and is autoimmune, meaning that the immune system attacks cells in the pancreas just as it would a virus or bacteria. The tendency is inherited with a 50 percent concordance in identical twins. The person with this type of diabetes will always be dependent upon insulin injections.

Type II diabetes usually begins in adulthood. It is inherited, but not autoimmune. There is 100 percent concordance in identical twins. Degeneration of the pancreas is accelerated and insulin reserves become inadequate. Insulin treatment is not usually required in early stages, and maybe not ever. The disease can be controlled with diet, exercise, and stress management. Some cases have been brought into remission through the use of nutribionic treatment — tissue regeneration. Insulin treatment may become necessary as the process advances with time. Ten percent of all 80-year-olds will have some degree of Type II diabetes.

Alice developed diabetes in her late 50s. She had been feeling tired, and generally not well. She could never seem to satisfy her thirst, and often drank three or four glasses of water at a time. Then she would void it all out in just a few minutes. The doctor thought at first that the disease could be controlled by diet and exercise, which is often the case in Type II diabetes.

But even following the doctor's orders, Alice's blood sugar continued to skyrocket to 500 or more (normal range is 65 to 115). Medication failed, as well. A specialist in diabetes, an endocrinologist, put her on insulin. At first, she would have reactions to the insulin and her blood sugar would drop too low. However, Alice is a person who intelligently monitors her body, following a self-care regimen in order to stay well. She tests her blood sugar three times a day. She follows a diabetic diet and eats at regular intervals. She has learned how to balance the timing of food, exercise, and insulin. Most importantly, she is alert to signals from her body that help her avoid crises. Alice, at the age of 70, runs three miles every morning of the year. She runs outside in the summer, spring, and fall, and in the winter she runs around her church gym. She has made a decision to take care of her health.

Musculoskeletal System

Healthy bone is very hard living tissue, supplied with nutrients and hormones carried by the blood. The center of the bone, the **marrow** (not pictured), makes red cells for the blood. There are about 230 bones in the body. Some of them give the body shape and support; others protect softer parts of the body. For example, the skull protects the brain, which is very soft and vulnerable to injury. The ribs protect the heart and lungs.

The outer layer of bone is hard, but just underneath is a spongy layer, and the marrow is in the center. Bones are always connected by **joints**, some of which are very mobile, as in your elbow or knee. Others have minimal motion, like the ribs, and still others have virtually no mobility, as in the skull. Over the outside of the bone is a thin, thready layer, the periosteum. In a disease like osteoporosis, the hard bone begins to get spongy, too, and breaks easily.

The movement of the joints and bones is controlled by **muscles**. Some, the flexors, are for bending, and some, the extensors, are for straightening. Cardiac muscle, and the smooth muscles in the uterus and intestinal tract, also contract and relax. Muscle fibers are able to shorten their length by 30 to 40 percent. Each muscle has a link to the nervous system. This allows information about the position and relative tension of a muscle to flow to the brain. The brain responds with instructions to the muscle to contract or relax. Hormones and chemicals play a part in how well these messages are sent and received. Around and between all parts of the body is connective tissue made of collagen.

At the beginning of this chapter, you read about Margaret and her fractured pelvis. When she was in traction, her muscles were not used for a while and became weak and stiff. A large part of Margaret's rehabilitation involved strengthening the unused muscles and obtaining mobility in the joints.

Immune System

If you like science fiction, you will love studying the immune system. It is complicated, fascinating, and mysterious. As was mentioned earlier, an army awaits inside you that is constantly on guard to protect you from disease-causing bacteria, from viruses, and from cancer. This army originates in your bone marrow, spleen, thymus gland, and lymph nodes. These organs and glands are like relay stations in your body. They communicate with each other and with the central nervous system. Messages are carried by means of chemicals circulating in the lymph and blood. These chemicals provide the triggers to activate the various arms of the immune system. Certain kinds of cells are released to fight off the aliens who have invaded your body.

Imagine this: you are working in your rose garden, and as you mix the bone meal into the soil around the bushes, you snag your finger on a thorn. You don't think much about it, although it did tear the flesh enough to bleed. You go on working because it looks like rain, and you want to finish the job. About 30 minutes later, you go into the house to wash. You notice that it is a nasty wound after all, but you don't have time to do much about it except to slap on a bandaid. The next morning your finger is red and slightly swollen. The day after that there seems to be quite a lot of pus forming in the wound, and the finger is painful. So you clean it up and apply an antibiotic ointment. On the third day, there is a red streak up the inside of your wrist and you have a headache. At that point, you decide to get medical help. As it turns out, you have a bacterial infection caused by organisms that entered your body from the soil. Fortunately, you receive treatment and recover.

This is what happened: when the bacteria entered your torn finger, they immediately began to multiply. Just as quickly, the patrol cells, called **lymphocytes**, which are wandering around checking things out, spot the bacteria and quickly report back to the lymph node headquarters that an enemy alien has entered the body. The lymphocytes are then transformed into **plasma cells**, which get busy manufacturing antibody proteins specific for that bacteria, pouring them rapidly into the bloodstream. These plasma cells are called **B-lymphocytes** because they were created in the bone marrow. Meanwhile, certain white cells called **phagocytes** try to destroy the bacteria. At the same time, a message is sent back to headquarters asking the chief to send help. **Macrophages** come to the rescue because they kill even more bacteria. In this war, they overcome and destroy many of the bacteria, but in the process they themselves are destroyed. The pus you see in your finger is made up of dead bacteria and dead white cells. The redness and swelling are evidence that the battle is going on. In the case of your wounded finger, it turned out to be a bigger battle than expected. **T-lymphocytes**, which are created in the thymus gland, transform themselves into mean, aggressive killer cells. These killers go to work in earnest to save your life. You also had help from your doctor, who prescribed antibiotics, because your immune system wasn't strong enough to win the battle alone.

In the case of your rose thorn wound, your immune system was unable to react strongly enough. It can also happen that your immune system will fail to react to abnormal growth of cells in your body, such as cancer cells. In reality, you may have cancer many times in your life, but your immune system is able to recognize and destroy it. If your immune system has become weakened, the cancer may be allowed to grow.

The immune system can become overly zealous and react too much to plant pollens, animal dandruff, or house dust, causing the sneezing, runny nose, itchy eyes, and coughing that spells allergy. It can even become severe enough to cause anaphylactic shock, which is life-threatening.

In some people, the immune system is misdirected, and attacks normal cells as if they were invaders. Then you are said to have an autoimmune disease, such as systemic lupus, rheumatoid arthritis, Type I diabetes, thyroiditis, or eczema. There is often a genetic factor involved in this wayward behavior of the immune system, and it is difficult to control. You do have a certain amount of control over the behavior of your immune system, as you will see later on.

If your immune system did not work at all, you would die. You've heard about children who live in plastic bubbles to protect them from infection. These children have no ability to fight infection, and even in a bubble they may die. AIDS is an example of failure of the immune system. In this case, a virus is the cause of this acquired immune deficiency.

The immune system is much more complicated than I have described. The field of immunology is one that is ripe for new discoveries. There is much yet to be learned, and you may enjoy reading some of the books listed in the reference section at the end of this chapter.

Brain and Nervous System

As complicated as the immune system is, its complexity is certainly matched by that of the brain and nervous system. Your heart can be kept beating by artificial means, and a machine can breathe for you. If your kidneys fail, another machine can perform their functions, but if your brain stops working, you're dead.

There are 10 billion **nerve cells** in the brain alone. Nerves from all over the body can transmit messages back to the brain, via the **spinal cord**, at a speed of 270 miles per hour. These transmissions are faster than the most sophisticated computer, and certainly much faster than making a telephone call. If a telephone call could be as fast as nerve transmission, the person you are calling would say "hello" before you picked up the phone to dial.

If you look in an anatomy book, you begin to get some idea of the complexity of the brain and nervous system. The expression "I'm nervous" strikes me as being obvious. Everyone is "nervous" in the sense that we all have nerves, and those nerves are busy sending messages all the time. Sometimes the messages are sent too fast or too slow, and occasionally the system fails so that some messages are not received — but everyone is "nervous"!

The **brain** has many different parts. The two major halves are called **cerebral hemispheres**, and that is where conscious thoughts, memory, and speech take place. The **cortex**, or outer layer of each hemisphere, does the work. In order for the brain to be contained within the skull, it is wrinkled and convoluted so that it can have maximum surface area. Brain size is not necessarily related to intelligence. It is said that the French philosopher Anatole France had a brain much smaller than average. Even when you are asleep, 50,000,000 nerve messages are relayed back and forth between the brain and different parts of the body every second.

Brain activity is primarily electrical. Electrical currents are sent from nerve cells in the brain to and from millions of nerve cells in the body. Nerve cell units are called **neurons**, and come in a variety of shapes and sizes. Each neuron, which measures about 0.025mm across, has a tiny electrical charge, even when not in use. This electrical charge is produced by the chemical difference between the interior of the nerve cell and the tissue surrounding it. Touching and tasting, for example, alter this chemical balance and cause an electrical change. This change triggers a series of similar changes along the length of the nerve fiber. It's like a spark along a fuse. Millions of neurones fire impulses every second. These messages are coded so that the brain can decide what instruction to send back. When the foot says, "Help me, I'm standing on a nail," and the hand says, "A fly is crawling on me," the brain will choose the most urgent signal and lift the foot first.

The brain keeps you alive by balancing the processes of growth and decay. It controls all the body's mechanisms. Your brain is what puts you in the driver's seat. It surveys all functions of the body simultaneously to ensure that all operations are coordinated. The brain is like an air traffic controller. The controller has to watch his radar screen and keep track of many planes all at once. Then he has to send messages to each one to keep them in their proper places so they won't fly into each other. The brain never takes a vacation. Even when injured, parts of the brain will compensate for the injured parts, unless the damage is too massive.

How you make decisions; what you dream, think, and feel; and how you behave are all functions of the brain. Most of this falls under your conscious control. This should reassure you — it means that you have control of yourself and your environment to a great degree. That is why I have saved this discussion of the brain for the end of the chapter. You have access to more information about your inner systems than you probably have ever imagined. I believe that when you learn to monitor these systems, and develop an automatic awareness of their state of being, you can control 80 percent of threatening illnesses and maintain a desirable state of health. Sometimes amazing things can happen, as you will see in the following case.

Tom and Leah

I am acquainted with a young man who, in his first year of medical school, was diagnosed with leukemia. His doctors wanted to give him a chemical treatment which would have rendered him sterile. Tom and Leah had married during the previous summer and had plans for a family. Against the advice of professors, doctors, family, and friends, Tom refused to receive chemotherapy. Through a deep state of relaxation, Tom was able to achieve heightened bodily awareness. He was able to sense what was happening with the malignant cells in his blood. Over the next several months, he practiced visualizing these cells, manipulating them in various fanciful ways. He communed with his immune system, guiding it in the direction of healing. Even though he felt ill much of the time, Tom stayed in school.

His teachers thought his career was doomed. At the end of six months, he was feeling better and his blood had reverted to normal. That was 12 years ago. That young man is practicing psychiatry today, and his doctors are still waiting for him to relapse. It was an incredible accomplishment that demonstrated the power of the human mind.

Inner Systems Inventory

The aim of this chapter has been to focus your attention on the wondrous living systems inside you. Perhaps this last section has taught you things you didn't know about your different physical systems and their interrelationships. Perhaps the coloring exercise gave you insight into your own emotional awareness of these processes. Both types of information are vital steps toward taking charge of your health.

This book is not about curing cancer. It is not going to recommend that everyone who has cancer should refuse chemotherapy. Rather, it is about being in control of your own life: knowing what is happening to you at every level — from the microscopic to the universal — and improving what you can. In the next chapter, you begin to learn about controlling the world around you. But first, it makes sense to stop and assess the current state of your health.

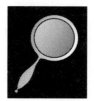 And here is your next exercise: a real-life one. If you have not had a medical checkup recently, now is a good time. Take with you the Living Systems Inventory, *Inner Systems*, on the next page, and ask the doctor to check the assets and liabilities for each category. The chart is organized in a way the doctor will understand: from vital systems to supporting systems. It makes use of a "balance sheet" analogy, just as in financial bookkeeping. Of course, the resources being assessed here are more precious.

When you are at your doctor's, ask for copies of lab, x-ray, and other diagnostic reports. Keep these in a three-ring binder. You can add to them every time you have tests of any kind. Always place the newest one on top. The doctor only needs to do the checklist once. After that you can record what you learn in an office visit yourself. If you should be hospitalized, get and keep copies of tests, discharge summaries, and bills. Your doctor may charge for a longer visit the day he fills out the form, but it's worth it.

For an example, look at the inventory Meredith had her doctor fill in. Meredith is an energetic woman in her 60s who has been generally healthy all her life. She decided to schedule her annual physical early this year because of problems she was having with her right knee. Lately, as she did her daily five-mile bike ride, her knee began to feel painful, and now it was swollen as well. She used this opportunity to have her doctor fill out her Inner Systems Inventory.

Sometimes, I'm sorry to say, older people are not listened to with as much respect as younger patients. Even sadder is the fact that women's statements about symptoms are disregarded more frequently than are those made by men. You and I can change that by being informed. We can ask questions, and we can present evidence from our notebooks if we seem to not be believed. At each visit, ask about your blood pressure and make note of the numbers for your own record.

These documents are extremely valuable if your doctor moves away, or you have to go to a new doctor. When the old doctor says he will send your records to the new one, he doesn't mean the whole chart; he means a summary letter and some lab reports. The letter is usually brief and fairly often inaccurate. That's just one of the liabilities of the medical system. These overworked, harassed men and women just don't have time to be thorough. They rely on their memories too much. It's no use being angry about it; just take control of your medical care by keeping your own records. If a doctor wants to see some of your records, give him copies, and keep your copies. If your present doctor is unwilling to participate with you in this kind of team effort, get a new doctor.

Living Systems Inventory

Inner Systems

Your Name: _____   *Date:* _____

Physician: _____

System	Asset	Liability	Action (medical; therapeutic)
Brain and Nervous			
Cardiovascular			
Respiratory			
Digestive			
Bladder and Kidneys			
Endocrine			
Reproductive			
Musculoskeletal			
Immune			

Specific instructions: _____

_____

_____

Tests Ordered:_____

Test Results: _____

Other Physicians Consulted: _____

Living Systems Inventory

Inner Systems

Your Name: Meredith Lamm

Physician: A. Carlise, M.D.

System	Asset	Liability	Action (medical; therapeutic)
Brain and Nervous	Mental status and neurological OK.	No liability.	None.
Cardiovascular	Heartbeat strong/ regular. No sign of arterial disease.	Blood pressure 180/110.	Monitor 3 days & report.
Respiratory	Breath sounds normal — no rates.	No liability.	Continue conditioning excercise program.
Digestive	Normal bowel sounds.	Complains of "heartburn."	Antacids 2 weeks and report.
Bladder and Kidneys	Urinalysis OK — no complaints	No liability.	None.
Endocrine	Thyroid, ovaries normal size.	Blood glucose 140.	None.
Reproductive	Hysterectomy 10 yrs ago.	No liabilities.	None.
Musculoskeletal	Muscle strength and tone OK.	Right knee swollen, stiff, painful.	Ice pack for pain. X-ray.
Immune	Rarely ill.	No apparent liability-except arthritis?	None now. Check rheumatoid factor, ANA, compliment.

Specific instructions: <u>Reduce Sodium intake, monitor blood pressure 3 days and report.</u>
<u>If knee pain does not yield to ice, call for x-ray report and possible additional lab tests.</u>

Tests Ordered: <u>Fasting-Glucose tolerance; x-ray right knee.</u>

Test Results: <u>Pending</u>

Other Physicians Consulted: <u>None at present.</u>

References

Bender, D.L., and B. Leone, series eds. (1990) *The Elderly: Opposing Viewpoints*. San Diego, CA: Greenhaven Press.

Bisacre, M., ed. (1979) *The Human Body and How It Works Illustrated Encyclopedia*. New York: Exeter Books.

Burns, G. (1983) *How To Live to be 100 — or More*. New York: G.P. Putnam and Sons.

Fekete, I., and P.D. Ward (1984) *The World of Science: Your Body*. New York: Facts on File Publications.

Gamlin, L. (1988) *The Human Body*. New York: Gloucester Press.

Miller, J.G. (1978) *Living Systems*. New York: McGraw-Hill Book Company.

Nourse, A. (1982) *Your Immune System*. New York: Franklin Watts.

The Rand McNally Atlas of the Body and Mind (1976) Mitchell Beazely Publications, Ltd.

2

Your Outer Systems

In this chapter, you will turn your focus to the larger systems of which you are a part: the world around you. Although these outside resources and supports are physically outside of you, they are an integral part of you — surrounding, embracing, and working for and with you. Your family and friends can give as much life support as your own inner resources do.

An unborn baby lives in a protected environment. His internal systems are still developing and have not yet experienced the great demands that will later be placed upon them. His world is small. He is a completely dependent being, relying upon his mother's body to perform vital functions. Her decisions about food, rest, and activity determine his health.

You are a little bit like that unborn child. Of course you are independent in the sense that you are not connected umbilically to any life-sustaining entity. But how independent are you, really? Where do you get food? How do you heat your living space? Obvious questions, but important, because a vital step to maintaining control of your life is to understand your interdependency with other systems, your physical environment, and relationships with people.

Margaret, the woman who suffered the broken pelvis in Chapter 1, found she had to stretch her arms out to family, friends, and beyond for support in her recovery. What is your posture toward your environment? Are you reaching out, or turning away? A look at the world outside yourself begins with you, for that is where the contact comes from.

Personal and Family Inventories

Yourself

When you draw up a balance sheet at the end of the year, you are faced with this problem: what is asset and what is liability? Your shiny new car is an asset, but it is also a liability because your insurance rates are higher than they were for the old car. That

Christmas bonus was a wonderful asset at the time, but do you now have to pay taxes on it? In a similar way, people can be both asset and liability, too.

 On the following pages you will gradually put together a family balance sheet, if you will. Here you can evaluate your own and your family's assets and liabilities. You'll begin with one person — yourself — and one category — assets — to get a feel for this. Later you'll have a chance to consider liabilities, and to apply the same process to people around you. On the Living Systems Inventory, *Myself,* list yourself by name, and begin to write down your personal assets. An asset is anything you like about yourself, such as appearance, character traits, things you have accomplished, ambitions you may have for the future, and skills you have developed. Rack your brain and come up with as much as you can.

Sometimes people have a hard time getting started because it is not the usual thing to be thinking about — how wonderful you are. You were probably taught to do just the opposite. One way to start is to ask someone you trust what she or he sees in you that is admirable. That will stimulate your thinking in the right direction. Be sure to leave room for the assets you will think of later.

If you have difficulty thinking of words to describe your behaviors, attitudes, and personal characteristics, you may find help in the following list. Your words are better than mine, so use this list only as a way to stimulate thinking.

Assets Starter List

Compassionate	Kind	Responsible	Stubborn
Good at art	Like music	Good mother	Inquisitive
Speak languages	Read a lot	Homemaker	Good listener
Relaxed	Compulsive	Attractive	Intelligent
Expressive	Affectionate	Friendly	Nice hair
Businessman	Solve problems		Neighborly

Once you've made an initial list of personal assets, you'll want to balance them by considering personal liabilities. You probably don't need suggestions for liabilities. Most people have little difficulty in thinking about their faults. Liabilities would include habits, behaviors, physical details, and attitudes you don't like about yourself. Be honest in completing the liabilities list: these are things you want to acknowledge so you can work to change some of them. After you have listed liabilities, go back and think about your assets again. Some of your assets may also be liabilities, or the other way around.

For example, Lee had many more assets than he recognized at first. All of his working years were spent farming. He was a successful farmer. He was able to provide for his family and send three sons and two daughters to college. From the time his oldest boy was ready for 4-H, Lee was right there with him, involved in the boy's projects and teaching crop management to an older group. One year he was chosen "Farmer of the Year" in Iowa. Lee didn't think of any of those things as assets until his wife pointed them out.

Living Systems Inventory

Myself

Your Name: _____

Assets	Liabilities

"I was just doing what was there to be done," Lee said.

"Isn't that an asset?" Martha asked, "Some don't do what needs to be done."

Lee had to admit this was true, and reluctantly wrote it all down. Then he hesitated. "That 'Farmer of the Year' thing might not be an asset," he said.

"Whyever not?" demanded Martha. "I don't see just anyone getting that."

"I know, I know, Martha, but think about those times when I had to go out of town."

"Well, that was part of the job," Martha said.

"Yeah, but Roy got into trouble that one time because I wasn't here to handle him."

"We don't know for sure you could've stopped him. You probably could, but it doesn't matter now. Just list 'Farmer of the Year' as both asset and liability."

"Oh," said Lee in surprise, "I guess it was both good and bad, wasn't it?"

Connie, whose partial inventory is shown below, noticed that an asset, such as perfectionism, can be both asset and liability. Her home always looked nice, but her over-concern about neatness was annoying to others. Seeing this spelled out in black and white was like reading pages from her own mind. Organizing things in this way gave her the beginning of control. In her assets list, she saw what resources she'd have to draw on; and in her liabilities list, she saw what things she'd like to change.

It will be interesting for you to see what happens as a result of this kind of organization. Most likely you will find that you — like every other person — have some behaviors, attitudes, and personal characteristics that may be annoying to others and are, therefore, liabilities. Since no one person has only liabilities, you will find that you have your fair share of assets, too.

After organizing your impressions in this way, you need to leave it alone for a time to let your deeper mind work. When you finally get to the problem-solving stage, you'll find that your list of assets suggests many personal resources. You'll want that list of assets to be as complete as possible; so allow yourself time to reflect and come back to it. That's the way your mind works. It will do its job if you give it a chance.

Living Systems Inventory

Myself

Connie

Assets	Liabilities
Neat, perfectionistic about work.	Drive other people crazy with neatnik behavior.
Friendly.	Family cannot relax in my house.
Like to read and paint.	Wear myself out trying to be perfect.
Look OK for 75.	
Feel good about my past life.	

Your Family

On the Living Systems Inventory, *Family*, (next page) list each person in your family. Then start thinking about and listing their assets and liabilities just as you did for yourself. There may be a person in your family whose behavior and personality are so irritating to you that he or she seems to be a total liability. List all of that person's liabilities; think about them and try to be fair. Then, as you begin to list assets, try hard to be fair about that, too. Most people have some good qualities. It is important to recognize the liabilities, and equally important to know the assets. Perhaps you can use an asset to balance a liability in the same person. If cousin Charley's only asset is a nice smile, you have a tool for changing your relationship with Charley and at the same time helping Charley to grow. You do that by complimenting Charley on his nice smile every time you see him. It is also helpful if you can comment on Charley's nice smile when you are talking to others. Charley may never change all of his bad habits, so you have a choice: you can either accept Charley with all of his faults or you can let that relationship go and spend your energy improving more promising relationships.

People who are no longer living belong on your family chart, too. If you think about the deceased, even occasionally, no matter how long they have been dead, then you still have a relationship with them and they need to be included. Certainly there are people in my life that I remember and some that I think about often. Sometimes I even write letters to them in my journal. Your deceased people have assets and liabilities that still affect you today. The very absence of their living presence affects you. It's all part of your living systems network — you support others and they you. You are part of the fabric of each other's lives, even after death.

What follows is part of Connie's family inventory. Can you find possibilities for change and growth in the assets and liabilities she listed for her son and daughter?

Living Systems Inventory

My Family

<u>Connie</u>

Person & Relationship	Assets	Liabilities
Son: Don	Loving, kind, cares about family. Makes do with little $. Spends time with family.	Never been organized. Lacks ambition...doesn't stay in any job long.
Daughter: Susan	Smart. Pres. of the corporation... Makes $$$. Beautiful. Perfectionist like me. Appreciates cultural things.	Too busy to pay attention to family. Divorced. Doesn't spend enough time with her kids. I haven't seen her in a year.

Living Systems Inventory

My Family

Your name: _____

Person & relationship	Assets	Liabilities

It's important to understand these assets and liabilities in yourself as well as in others. You have no hope of changing something you can't define. Connie still has a chance to spend more time with her daughter. It's not too late to be a friend to the grandchildren. She can make decisions now and take action to change her own behaviors and attitudes. By so doing, Connie may change how her daughter and her daughter's family relate to her.

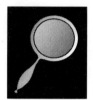
When you have thoroughly evaluated every family member, think about how they are located spatially in relationship to you. How close are you to one another emotionally? Perhaps you live in Los Angeles and your son in Denmark. It could be that the distance in miles is not terribly important if you have frequent contact and if you have an emotional bond. On the other hand, your brother may live two blocks away and yet be so distant emotionally that it is as if he didn't exist. This exercise gives you another way of looking at your current family situation.

Anita, for example, has varying distances from her family. Anita has had a hard life. Her first husband, an alcoholic, left her with four children after 15 years of a miserable marriage. She has a nicer husband now, but she knows where the old one is and hears from him occasionally. Two of her daughters graduated from college and are managing both family and career. They don't have much time for Anita, although they keep in touch. Another daughter, a high school dropout, keeps herself anonymous most of the time. Maybe twice a year she calls to pour out her heart and express love and appreciation for her mother. This daughter is much in her mother's thoughts. Anita's son is a real estate broker in the town where Anita lives. He lives on the other side of town, but then Greenspring isn't all that big. He is very busy. Once a month, on a Sunday afternoon, he brings his family for a formal afternoon visit. They wear their best clothes, and perch uncomfortably, eating cookies Anita has prepared for their visit. They seem to have a hard time thinking of things to say. The teenage grandchildren look bored, and give each other rolling-eyed looks that clearly say, "When are we gonna get outa here?" They have never responded to Anita's grandmotherly overtures, and she is as glad to have them go as they are to leave. Anita's husband doesn't have much use for this scene, so he usually goes for a walk.

Anita decided to draw a diagram of her family, arranging it to represent both spatial and emotional distance. On the following page, you can see what she drew. It's interesting that Anita chose different-sized circles to represent individuals in her family. It's not hard to tell that she has never developed a relationship with her daughter-in-law, is it? And what happened to the sons-in-law? They aren't even present!

Use the blank space below Anita's drawing to sketch a diagram of your own family relations. As you draw your family, be as creative as you like. Use stick men, circles, squares, and triangles...whatever you feel like doing. Remember that these are subjective impressions — and, of course, that no one need see your own drawing but you.

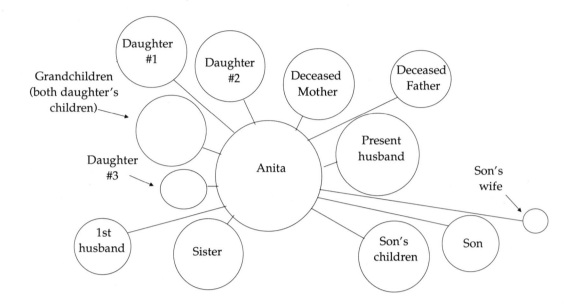

As you were doing this exercise, you probably became aware that it isn't always clear how close or distant people are. There may be qualities about a person that make you feel close, and other things that make you feel distant. You may have had to think a bit and weigh the degree of closeness before you could draw. Everyone has good qualities and bad habits. Everyone is both nice and naughty. Everyone is, at the same time, generous and selfish.

Anita's son and his family are assets, because she loves them. Their liability is that they have not tried to nurture and develop relationships with Anita. On the other hand, Anita's liability may be that she has not done all she could do to foster family feeling.

Daughter number 3 represents a liability because Anita never knows where she is, and she worries constantly about what kind of life she is living. Nevertheless, this daughter has many assets. Anita knows that her daughter loves and cares for her, but is unable to live in a traditional style. Anita knows, without any doubt, that if something bad happened, daughter number 3 would be at her side as fast as she could get there.

As you reflect on your family sketch, think about what you can add to the assets and liabilities columns in your family inventory. That will help you think about possibilities for change and growth in yourself, and in all your family relationships.

Friends

The Living Systems Inventory on the next page is to use for evaluating your friends. You know these people differently than you do family members. Usually you are not privy to personal knowledge of them from birth onward. Still, they are part of your personal world and support network. In many cases, friends share an intimacy as close, closer, or entirely different from actual family, and they can come to seem a separate, chosen family in your life. It's a good idea to include acquaintances on your inventory of friends as well, because anyone you know has an effect on your life, just as you do on theirs. It may even happen that a present acquaintance will someday become your friend. Please take plenty of time with this part of the assignment. Being thorough here will help you formulate a complete picture of your support network, a richer fabric than you may at first realize. It can be joyous to reflect on friendships, and to find opportunities to continue strengthening them.

Complete Living Systems Inventory

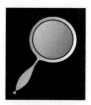 Now that you've had a chance to focus on separate levels of your living systems network — yourself, your family, your friends — it can be tremendously helpful to organize this information into an overview: a complete systems inventory. You'll have a chance to expand this overview still further in a later chapter, "Getting Involved." For now, it's enough to begin by looking over the separate inventories you've been working on.

Since you'll want to condense things a bit on your Complete Living Systems Inventory, here's an idea for focusing in still further. Look at each asset for each person you listed, and think about what those assets can *do* for you as well as for others. Maybe a nice smile can brighten a dreary day; maybe a penchant for neatness or literature can inspire you. Don't worry about "using" people for their assets; you'll have ample chance to pay back with your own assets! The idea is to find the *resources* available in each relationship all around you.

Your friends, your family, your neighbors — all might be valuable resources. Look back to your friend inventory to begin, and write the names of those most able to give and share on the Complete Living Systems Inventory at the end of this chapter. In the column next to their names list the assets you picked out from the friends inventory. Just to balance things out, you might jot down their main liabilities in the next column, Liabilities. But focus your attention on the Resources column. This is where you can translate assets into action. It's also where you can note tangible resources, like a car or a

Living Systems Inventory

My Friends

Your name: _____

Person	Assets	Liabilities

large private library. Put down what you can for each of your friends. Then, go ahead: write, in the next column, how you personally can benefit from these resources.

Next, look back to the liabilities column — it's time to even things out. Are there liabilities you can compensate for? Think about the friends you already listed. Whatever *you* can do for *them*, write in the final column. Also think about the friends you haven't yet listed. Could you help those people in any way? Add their names, their liabilities, and what you might do to help. Try, too, to add their assets to the list.

After Lila completed her inventory on friends, she saw that of all her friends, Jane and Gwen were particularly close. They had exhibited caring behavior in the past, and had many assets. Lila also recognized that her assets were uniquely useful to Jane and Gwen, and so the reciprocal relationship they had enjoyed in the past could be enhanced to mutual benefit. This is what the Resources and the two other columns next to it look like in Lila's complete inventory:

Next, you'll want to consider your family. Proceed just as you did with friends, looking back to your original inventory and listing assets, liabilities, resources, and ways you can help one another. Take all the time you need to consider your family.

Complete Living Systems Inventory

Lila

Systems	Resources	How this person/resource can help me	How I can help others
Friends:			
Jane	Drives, likes to shop.	Take me to Dr. and shopping.	Type her family notes.
Gwen	Good to talk to. Listens.	I can discuss problems.	Take care of her dog when she leaves town.

Finally, you'll want to return to yourself. From your personal inventory, add your own assets and liabilities to the complete list. Then use the same process you did for your family and friends to create resources from your assets. What can you do to help others? You started writing some ideas above — now you might expand those sections, too. Give yourself credit as a valuable resource to others.

Don't forget your inner systems. This is the most intimate level of the inventory, and you can think of it however you like. In Chapter 1, you considered your physical systems in detail, and noted assets and liabilities. Some of those ideas belong here. Can others help you deal with physical shortcomings? Can you use physical strengths, or experience in illness, as resources for helping others? This physical dimension is an important consideration. But you may also want to include such ideas as faith and knowledge under the inner systems category. It's your world.

Having a reciprocal network of support systems is insurance against loneliness and fear. If you have ever lived in a small town or rural area during the first half of the 20th century, you know how well that can work. It's just that nowadays, particularly in larger cities, you have to make your support system work for you. Each level of your living system is a resource and an opportunity. Anchored by family and friends, and strengthened by your own assets, you have ample resources to draw on as you face the challenges of life and the world. Chapter 9, "Getting Involved," will offer more ideas on reaching out to larger systems. In coming the chapters, you will see how you help create the world you live in, and you'll learn how you can work to shape that world.

References

Klass, P. (1987) *A Not Entirely Benign Procedure: Four Years as a Medical Student.* New York: G.P. Putnam and Sons.

Lewis, F.C. (1968) *Patients, Doctors, and Families.* Garden City, New York: Doubleday and Co., Inc.

Complete Living Systems Inventory

Your name: _____

System	Assets	Liabilities	Resources	How this person/resource can help me	How I can help others
Friends: _____ _____ _____					
Family: _____ _____ _____					
Myself:					
Inner Systems					

3

Thoughts, Feelings, and Behavior

If you are like most older people, what you fear is losing your independence. Dependence means not being able to live alone in your own space when you choose to. It means needing others to help you with cooking, cleaning, and — horror of horrors — bathing and dressing. It means not being able, or not being allowed, to make decisions about where you will live, what treatment you will receive, or who will take care of your money. Sometimes it even means not being allowed to decide what you would like for dinner, or even if you want dinner at all.

Loss of independence doesn't happen to everyone. Many people make it all the way to the end without giving up the right to make decisions and to care for themselves. You can't predict whether you will be one of the lucky ones or not. What you can do is face the fear, define the needs, and make decisions *now*, while you can.

Inez

My mother, Inez, valued her independence fiercely. She had it all figured out that she would die in her sleep at home. The only flaw in her plan was that something unexpected might happen over which she would have no control. "What do you fear, mother?" I asked, on more than one occasion.

"A broken hip," she replied without hesitation. "I've seen it happen too many times around here." ("Here" was the retirement community in which she lived, in her own little cottage.) "They fall and break their hips, and then they don't last long after that."

"Some do," I said. "Look at Mr. Beasely. He had surgery and now he's OK."

"OK?" she said, in that how-can-you-even-think-such-a-thing voice. "He's in a nursing home. His children just came in and moved out all of his things. They only visit him once a week, and heaven only knows what atrocities are perpetrated upon him in the meantime." And so her fear became my fear.

We subscribed to a "Lifeline" service so that she could summon assistance by pressing the center of a medallion she wore around her neck. She didn't want it at first. To her it seemed like the first step to dependency. It was a good thing she had it.

One day the phone rang while I was in a session with a student. It was the hospital emergency room. "Your mother's lifeline alarm went off," the voice said, "and we get no response to our call-back."

"I'll go right over," I said, fear grasping my stomach.

There was no car available that day, but my student volunteered to give me a lift. As we drove into the parking lot, I saw a group of people gathered around someone on the ground in front of my mother's cottage. Leaping out of the car, I half-ran as fast as I could with my cane clunking along beside.

"I'm coming, mother," I yelled as we got nearer. I was terrified that those people would do the wrong thing. As I approached the group, one woman said, "We tried to help Inez get up, but she couldn't do it." Oh no, I thought, why didn't they just leave her alone?

My mother was lying on her back, obviously in pain, but maintaining her dignity and poise all the same. When I asked where it hurt, she laid her hand on her left groin, and I knew it had to be a hip. In the next few minutes, I called the Lifeline number to report the need for an ambulance, and made my mother as comfortable as possible. The ambulance appeared and the whole incident — from the time Inez pushed her button to the time she entered ER (the emergency room) — lasted 15 minutes. Without Lifeline I don't know how long it would have taken my mother's friends to find my number and make the call. This way ER was expecting her before I even called back. They were ready. The doctor said the speed with which we had gotten her into the hospital probably saved her from complications, such as a blood clot — a common problem with hip fractures.

Several years earlier, Inez had made a decision which eased the entire hospital process. She added my name and my sister's name to her checking and savings accounts so that we could take care of financial matters in an emergency. She discussed all of her affairs and her wants and wishes with us, so we felt fairly certain we were doing right. Inez was 85 when she made that decision.

The sad thing was that this accident was the very thing Inez feared most. I think her conviction that a person couldn't recover from a broken hip hastened her demise. Although the surgery went well, and the hospital course was uneventful, her transfer to a rehab hospital was disastrous. To her it looked like a nursing home. She rapidly lost strength, stopped eating, and died two weeks later. Her belief prevented her from recovering, I think, and I just wish I had understood that better at the time.

What you believe, what you think, and what you feel cause you to behave in certain ways. The quality of life you lead from here on out is largely dependent upon what you think, what you say to yourself, and what decisions you make. You are not stuck with patterns of negative thinking. You need not lose hope of making things different. By assessing now where your fears and disappointments lie, you can begin to defeat them. Recognizing and acknowledging these perceptions is the first step.

How You Feel About Yourself

When you think about the times when you have felt unusually sad or very happy, what do you think caused those feelings? Do you believe your feelings were caused by what other people did or said, or by events that happened? Or do you believe your feelings came from inside you, from something you said or thought about? Now is your chance to discover more about your feelings and behaviors and what causes them.

Personal Assessment Scale

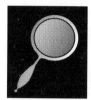 On the following page you will find a Personal Assessment Scale. This form is designed to help you review the attitudes that affect your mental and physical health. No one need see the form but you, and there are no "right" answers. What matters is that you are honest with yourself in completing it. Once you're done, your answers can show you which areas of your life you'd like to change. The changes may be in your thinking, in your behavior, or in your environment. For now, enjoy this opportunity for focused self-reflection.

Look over your responses to the Personal Assessment Scale to see where you stand. Remember that these are your own perceptions about yourself. If you circled numbers at the low end of the scale, you've had some experience making changes to adapt to new situations. If your numbers are on the high end of the scale, you'll face more challenges now, and your commitment will require more thought and stronger effort. But your rewards may be all the greater.

Scan your assessment to identify all areas where your answers were above four. Chances are you had a specific reason or issue in mind which led to your negative response. In the spaces below, you have an opportunity to briefly explain your reasoning for your response in each of these areas. You can respond to any of the categories you like. Of course, you'll want to pinpoint your problems in the problem areas. What led you to have these perceptions? These will be the areas for you to concentrate on, and you'll come back to them later. For now, just write what comes to mind.

Health

Many factors contribute to your health — physical, emotional, environmental, and psychological, to name a few. Which factors have led to your current state of wellness? You've experienced pain many times in your life, and you've recovered. Which factors have contributed to your return to wellness? For some people, psychological strength is the key; for others, a change in environment is more healing than a physical "cure." Think about things that have improved your health and things that have improved your perception of your health. Perhaps these things can be resources now.

Self-Assessment Level ___ Reasoning: _____

_____

_____

Personal Assessment Scale

1. **Health**: My perception of my general physical strength and wellness is:

1	2	3	4	5	6	7
Excellent						*Poor*

2. **Self-Image**: The image I have of myself as a person is:

1	2	3	4	5	6	7
Good						*Poor*

3. **Self-Fulfillment**: I believe that my wants and needs are satisfied:

1	2	3	4	5	6	7
Completely						*Not at all/rarely*

4. **Overall Feelings**: Most of the time I feel:

   4a. Anxiety

1	2	3	4	5	6	7
Secure						*Frightened*

   4b. Sadness

1	2	3	4	5	6	7
Happy						*Sad*

   4c. Anger

1	2	3	4	5	6	7
Serene						*Angry*

5. **Expectations**: I expect my future life to be:

1	2	3	4	5	6	7
Bright						*Cloudy*

6. **Interpersonal Relationships**: My relationships with others are:

1	2	3	4	5	6	7
Rewarding (Love)						*Conflicted (Hate)*

7. **Environmental Stresses**: The stresses in my life are:

1	2	3	4	5	6	7
Manageable						*Overwhelming*

8. **World Outlook**:

1	2	3	4	5	6	7
Good						*Grim*

Self-Image

What do you see in your mirror? Does it differ from the "you" others describe? How you see yourself affects every move you make, and every mood you feel. Perhaps you have ideas about yourself that have remained unchanged since childhood. Perhaps you exaggerate the changes life has brought you. You want to be as realistic in your appraisal of yourself as you are of others. Seeing yourself realistically means recognizing that you have pleasing attributes as well as a few imperfections. Give yourself a break! Life becomes harder than it needs to be when you see yourself as inadequate.

Self-Assessment Level ___ Reasoning: _____

_____

_____

Self-Fulfillment

Everyone has basic needs for food, water, shelter, and love. Nearly everyone desires more than the basics, such as education, entertainment, useful work, and so on. The degree to which you are satisfied with the way these needs and wants are being met influences your ability to take charge of your life.

Self-Assessment Level ___ Reasoning: _____

_____

_____

Overall Feelings

Just as with health, your feelings are influenced by many factors — both internal and external. These factors can seem unchangeable until you realize how much your *reaction* to and *interpretation* of events determine your feelings. You have probably looked at the same set of events twice, and reacted once with joy and optimism, and once with a feeling of doom.

Much of this chapter will focus on helping you recognize those reactions and take control of your feelings. Feelings are your direct line into your internal state. Behind most feelings are specific thoughts you can learn to hear. Chronic painful feelings are the prime evidence that you are engaging in unproductive, even harmful patterns of thought. How would you characterize your feelings? What issues came to mind when you first marked your levels on the self-assessment scale?

Anxiety *Self-Assessment Level* ___ Reasoning: _____

_____

_____

Sadness *Self-Assessment Level* ___ Reasoning: _____

_____

_____

Anger   *Self-Assessment Level* ___ Reasoning: _____

_____

_____

Expectations

The attitude you have developed about your future reveals how confident and optimistic you are. If you are convinced that nothing good will ever happen, and you tend to "awfulize" about things, then you probably also believe that whatever you do isn't going to make anything better. You can change your expectations and become more confident and optimistic by changing the way you talk to yourself. Instead of saying, "Everything's downhill from now on," you could say, "Things will work out if I just do the best I can for today." More about the value of positive self-talk is coming up.

Self-Assessment Level ___ Reasoning: _____

_____

_____

Interpersonal Relationships

How do you get along with others? Do you feel close to your family and friends, or are your relationships marked by conflicts that keep you from loving feelings? Most conflicts with family or close friends arise out of resistance to change. How true is this for you? Remember the role of other people in your Living Systems Inventory? How strong a support are they now? Where do you fit in *their* Living Systems Inventory?

Self-Assessment Level ___ Reasoning: _____

_____

_____

An anonymous poet offered this thought about relationships:

> I have wept in the night
> For the shortness of sight
> That to somebody's need made me blind;
> But I never have yet
> Felt a tinge of regret
> For being a little too kind.

Environmental Stresses

The stresses in your life measure the impact of unpleasant events that test your coping capabilities. Financial hardship, illness, loss of a loved one, war, drought, floods...the list is long of stressful things that can happen to you. Some people can take disasters in stride, others have a more difficult time.

How you cope is really dependent upon three things: what you say to yourself, what you do, and how you get involved with others in solving the problem. What stresses came to mind when you marked your self-assessment level? How have you responded to them?

Self-Assessment Level ___ Reasoning: _____

_____.

_____

World Outlook

This has to do with your perception of the character of your environment, including the larger world. The same world looks different to everybody, depending on individual perception and interpretation. What world events are on your mind these days? Do you see cause for hope in them, or for despair? Whether you focus on events in the news or on personal memories and contacts across the globe, your outlook on these larger systems can tell you something about your expectations for your own future. After all, the world is part of your personal living system.

Self-Assessment Level ___ Reasoning: _____

_____

_____

Thought Patterns

The above excerise led you to record some of your inner thoughts. If you look over your reasoning statements, you'll have a window into your distinctive patterns of thinking. It's just possible that there are patterns in your thinking, patterns which affect the way you perceive and process reality. By becoming aware of those patterns, you can begin to change the way you think and even feel about the same external circumstances. Below are eight typical patterns of thinking that can negatively affect your emotional well-being. (Adapted from *Thoughts and Feelings*, by McKay, Davis, and Fanning.) Do any look familiar to you?

1. Filtering

If you distort your thinking by the process of filtering, you magnify and "awfulize" your thoughts. Even though good things have happened to you, you tend to screen out the positive things and focus only on negative experiences. This kind of thinking makes everything seem more awful than it really is.

For example, a music teacher lost some of his students to a younger man. Under *Interpersonal Relationships*, he gave himself a "6." His reasoning went: "I am no longer a good teacher. I have alienated my students and lost my most rewarding human contact." Even though he had received compliments from other teachers...and even though many good students remained...he didn't remember these nice statements and relationships. He also failed to recognize the affection and regard from his family and nonprofessional friends.

Words that let you know you are filtering are: "terrible...awful...disgusting...horrendous," and so on. Do you see any of these words in your reasoning statements?

2. Polarized Thinking

This is black-and-white thinking: things must be all wrong or all right, all good or all bad, completely stupid or always smart. If you think this way, you can't allow yourself or others to make mistakes. Nothing can ever be average, and you find it hard to change your mind once you have made it up. An 85-year-old woman was constantly critical of herself because she didn't remember things as well as she used to. Under *Self-Image* she described herself as "dumb and completely useless."

3. Overgeneralizing

Words that let you know when you are overgeneralizing are: all, every, none, never, always, everybody, and nobody. Your children were good at that when they were small: "Everybody else gets to go to the circus...You never let me do anything...All the other girls have new dresses." The ways you overgeneralize now might be "I always forget to put out the trash...Nobody wants to spend time with an old woman...Every time I put on a clean blouse, I spill something on it." These are absolute statements that cause you to believe that you have no power to do differently. This kind of thinking puts you in a cage. Look for the tell-tale absolute words in your reasoning statements. Under *Anger*, one man wrote: "Of course I'm *always* angry. *Nobody* listens to what I say, and so I have to do *everything* myself."

4. Mind Reading

A mind reader is very judgmental. You try to figure out what the other person is thinking and then make assumptions about his or her behavior. When your children stop in for a hurried visit, you may think, "They only come because they have to, or because they don't want to hurt my feelings. They don't want to come here." Mind reading is often a case of assuming that others feel the same way you do, or that they will react to things the way you do. If you think in a suspicious way about how people treat you, then you think others think this way, too. Mind readers hardly ever bother to find out what the other person really is thinking or feeling. Check especially under Interpersonal *Relationship*s for evidence of mind reading.

5. Catastrophizing

Catastrophic thoughts often start with the words "what if." When a storm is predicted, you may refuse to go to lunch with your friend because you are saying, "What if I fall and break my hip?" A bout of diarrhea makes you fear colon cancer. When you read the obituaries, you wonder if you're next. And so it goes, on and on, your imagination feeding your fearful thoughts.

Catastrophizing stops you from seeing a situation as it is; instead, you project many steps forward into the worst possible future. It doesn't allow any room for positive, constructive action to change that future. And it doesn't let you enjoy the noncatastrophic present.

Fertile imaginations have a good time catastrophizing. Of course, they could have a better time applying their creative energies to solving present problems. Look especially under *Expectations* and *World Outlook* for signs that you dwell on worst possible cases.

6. Personalization

Personalization is the tendency to relate everything around you to yourself. A man went to the doctor for an annual checkup, and the doctor said that he'd like to be outside in the spring sunshine. The man thought the doctor meant it was a pain and a trial to have to be indoors doing his examination.

People who personalize are constantly comparing themselves to others: "She's older than I am but she doesn't show her age (I do)...He's not a good speaker (I am)...They saved money early in life (I didn't)." If you think in this manner, you are constantly questioning your worth. You use comparisons as a means to test your value. One man's response to *Self-Fulfillment* was a measure of how much less he had accomplished than his brother. When you come out better you feel superior, and that makes you even more judgmental. If you come out second best, you will indulge in envy and jealousy, both destructive feelings.

7. Blaming

Blaming involves making someone else responsible for choices and decisions that are actually your responsibility. A man got angry because his wife didn't mail the tax return. It wasn't really her problem; he hadn't told her it was ready to go. He expected her to read his mind. He rated his environmental stresses as high, but included in his reasoning many things he might have taken control of, such as seeing no flowers in his yard (he might have planted some) and hating the music his neighbor played (he might have complained, or played his own music).

If you're in the habit of blaming, you avoid the uncomfortable feelings that come with making a mistake. You can also indulge in self-pity because others are always making your life miserable. At our house we use blaming as a joke. If I spill a glass of water, I say to my husband, "It's all your fault," and laugh. We both know who spilled the water. When Walt burns the toast, he says, "You did it," and we laugh. We began to do that a long time ago when we needed to overcome the destructive thought pattern of blaming. Making a joke out of it helped us to do that. Blaming can also take the form of self-blaming. Usually, this is either a "Personalization" or a "Should." One woman said: "Things would've worked out better for me if I didn't have such a rotten personality. I should just stay home and not expose people to my unhappiness."

8. Shoulds

If you have inflexible rules about how you and other people should act, you may be a should-thinker. Since your rules are absolutely correct, you are in a position to find fault. This makes you irritable because people don't act right or think right. When others deviate from your values and standards, they are unacceptable and hard to be around. If your husband really loved you, he would send you flowers — as that is the right thing to do. If your children were not so selfish, they would ask you to dinner on Sundays. That is what they should do. Should, ought, and must are words that litter the speech of the should-thinker. "I know I should be happy and grateful," wrote one woman for a high measure of *Sadness*, "but I feel I should have done so much more with my life."

Should-thinkers apply these rules to themselves, too. Do any of these statements sound familiar?

> I must not become angry.
> I should be able to stand pain without complaining.
> I should never make mistakes.
> I ought to do more for my neighbors.
> I should be totally self-reliant.
> I should baby-sit the grandchildren more often.
> I must be a patient grandmother.
> I should always be serene and calm.
> I should love my children equally.
> I should have answers to everyone's problems.

Look over your reasoning statements in each category you assessed negatively. Do you see signs of any of these thought patterns? Identifying these thought patterns is the first step toward changing them. You might be able to recast them into more truthful and encouraging statements now. But thought habits are the result of a lifetime's conditioning, and it might take some work to spot and change them. You can learn to do it — and when you do, it will change the very quality of your feelings. The next section will help you through this process.

How You Create Your Feelings

Students of human behavior agree that thoughts precede feelings and behaviors. I know a woman whose primary behavior is one of withdrawal and disengagement from social interactions. She behaves this way because she is sad and doesn't have a very good opinion of herself. "I'm ugly and useless. I should be dead," is what she once admitted to me. My goodness, just typing words like that makes me feel sad. Wilma is saying that stuff all day long. Is it any wonder she doesn't want to fix her hair, or go out, or try to get involved with her grandchildren? She watches soaps, and lives those lives in fantasy. Most of those lives are pretty depressing, from what little I've seen.

Do you have negative thoughts? Do you talk to yourself in a depressing way? It's easy to do, isn't it? Everyone sometimes has difficulty maintaining positive self-talk. The great thing is, you can learn to spot this talk and change it to something better. When you learn to talk kindly to yourself, you will feel better, and then you will be able to take control of your life.

Spot and Stop Record

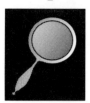

At first it is difficult to realize that feelings don't just arise spontaneously. They seem to, don't they? It may be hard to believe that the feelings did not come until after a negative thing you said to yourself, but I'm going to prove it to you. There are five steps to the following exercise. It will take more than a week to complete, but there is no need to stop reading here. The exercise can be an ongoing part of your day, every day.

Step 1

Make seven copies of the Spot and Stop Record on the next page.

Step 2

Each day, for a week, write down negative self-statements as they occur to you. These go in the first column, Spot.

When you wake up, check yourself out to see how you are feeling. Let's say you feel uneasy. Now stick with that uneasy feeling. Don't try to make it go away. See if you can identify what you were saying in your mind just a few seconds earlier. Was it something like, "Oh no, another day. How will I get through this day?" Or perhaps, "That backache is still there. I suppose it's going to hang around all day." Don't worry if you can't find the thought on this first try. It's hard at the beginning. Just get up and go about your morning routine, but keep your inner ear open for what you are saying. Eventually you will catch yourself saying something negative. When you do, write it in the first column of the Spot and Stop Record. Keep it handy so you can write on your chart throughout the day. At the end of the day, count up how many times you caught yourself being a negative self-talker. Do it again the next day, and the next, and the next, for a week. At the end of the week, you will be ready for the next task. Don't rush on, just stick with this assignment. It's an important building block.

Step 3

After a week of tracking negative self-talk, go back over your week's record. See if your thoughts contained words like "should," "have to," "ought to," "can't," or "must." So often this is the way people talk to themselves, as if a punishing or critical parent were lecturing.

Underline any words that sound like you are lecturing: shoulds, oughts, and so on. Look for blaming statements, global labeling, personalization, mind reading, filtering, or polarized thinking. Be on the lookout for catastrophizing. Then look for words that are clearly discouraging and self-demeaning, such as "I can't," "I never," and name-calling words.

Spot and Stop Record

(Make 7 copies)

Date:_____

Part A

Spot (Negative Self-Talk)	**Stop** (Negative Thought Patterns)	**Rational Comeback** (Healthy, Accurate Self-Talk)
_____	_____	_____
_____	_____	_____
_____	_____	_____
_____	_____	_____
_____	_____	_____
_____	_____	_____
_____	_____	_____
_____	_____	_____
_____	_____	_____
_____	_____	_____
_____	_____	_____
_____	_____	_____
_____	_____	_____
_____	_____	_____

Part B

My list of things, people, or events I enjoy: _____

_____

_____

_____

_____

_____

_____

Next, look for thoughts that dwell on worst cases, predictions of awful things about to happen, or of past events that were terrible. Have you heard yourself predicting failure during this past week? If you have, you have probably had feelings of anxiety, fear, and sadness. This kind of thinking can be called "awfulizing." It has also been called "ruminating," chewing the cud of awful thoughts. Any one of the thought patterns described earlier can show up in your negative self-talk. For now, it's enough just to recognize them. Write the negative thought patterns in the second column of the Spot and Stop Record.

Step 4

Circle the most frequent and painful examples of negative self-talk in your record. You'll want to compose rational comebacks to these statements. Below you'll find guidelines to help you do this in a systematic way. Your goal is to rewrite the statements to make them as accurate and healthy as possible. There is a place for your new statements in the third column of your Spot and Stop Record.

For example: Molly frequently said to herself, "Everything's downhill from now on. Getting old is the worst thing." Her new, healthy, accurate statement was, "Some days are easier than others. I can make a plan for getting through the tough days."

Below are some ways to talk back to yourself when you are using a particular negative thinking pattern. This is a handy reference section where you might want to place a permanent bookmark.

Rational Comebacks

1. Filtering

There are two things to do to get out of this pattern of focusing on things that upset you. First, *shift your focus to what action you can take to solve problems*. Say to yourself something like this, "It's OK, I can handle it," or "I've lived this long and managed pretty well, so I have a good track record of being able to cope with just about anything."

Second, *categorize the theme of your thinking*. Do your thoughts center on the losses you have experienced in life? Are you consumed with the unfairness of growing older? Do you dwell on being misunderstood? Balance this thinking by focusing on the opposite pole. Instead of loss, think of what you have gained from your life experiences. Replace thoughts of unfairness with plans for doing something to make someone else feel better. Rather than worrying about how others don't understand you, think about those who do. Or, as a project to explain yourself, write your personal history. You can come up with many ways to change your self-talk.

2. Polarized Thinking

The cure for this kind of thinking is simple: *stop making black-and-white judgments*. Almost nothing is completely terrible or completely wonderful, completely successful or completely a failure. No one is completely incompetent, no one has completely misspent his or her life. When you marked the Personal Assessment Scale, you placed yourself somewhere along a continuum. When you find yourself thinking in this black-and-white way, draw a straight line, label one end "good" or "right" or some other descriptive word, and the other end "bad" or "wrong." Then place yourself or the distressing event or the annoying person somewhere along that line. It is not realistic to say that a person is "wrong." He is some combination of wrong and right behaviors. And so are you.

3. Overgeneralization

You can change your tendency to exaggerate by following two steps. First, *monitor your vocabulary*. Avoid words that suggest extremes, like incredible, unbelievable, massive, awful, and so forth. Also watch out for "allness" words, such as every, all, always, never, everybody, and nobody. More appropriate words include: some, sometimes, and might.

Second, *test your self-talk by looking for evidence of truth in what you say*. You want to be as specific and accurate as possible. If you say "all," think of exceptions. If you say "most," think of numbers. If you can think of anything to refute your overgeneralized statement, you'll realize it was inaccurate.

4. Mind Reading

You can never know what someone else is thinking. I have been married for 42 years to the same man and he still surprises me with his thoughts. The cardinal rule here is *make no assumptions*. When you wonder what another person is thinking, you can do two things: you can ask, or you can test your assumptions by checking the evidence as you did for Overgeneralization. Asking is the best way.

5. Catastrophizing

How awful is it, really? To find out, *look for realistic odds*. If you think that you will inevitably die of cancer, check some statistics. Facts are readily available. What are the chances of your having colon cancer? Lung cancer? Prostate cancer? When, based on an honest evaluation of your risk factors, you see that your chances of having colon cancer are 30 percent, say to yourself, "That means I have a 70 percent chance of *not* having colon cancer. Those are good odds, and there are things I can do to prevent it."

Avoid absolute predictions about the future. If you continually say to yourself, "I'll die a sick and lonely old woman," you may be setting yourself up to do just that. The way you interact with others will be based on this prediction, and they will get the message to stay away. Instead, focus on the uncertainty of future events. There's as much room for hope as worry.

Finally, *avoid what ifs*. This line of thinking is bound to cause anxiety, because there is no way to predict or account for future possibilities. Only when your "what if" can lead to realistic problem solving (as in buying health insurance) is it a good idea to project worries into the future.

6. Personalization

Resist comparing yourself to someone else. Most comparisons are unfair. The one comparison you have a right to make is to yourself. It's fair to ask yourself, "Have I achieved the goals I set for myself this week?" It's quite all right to ask, "Am I improving in certain skills?" The only other fair comparison would be to someone who is identical to you in physical, mental, and emotional makeup and who has had exactly the same life experiences you have had. There is no such person. You are one of a kind. You have special attributes that are not like anyone else's.

7. Blaming

No one else is to blame for your unhappiness. You are not to blame for the unhappiness of another. Of course, sometimes things happen to you that you did nothing to provoke or deserve, such as robbery or abuse. It's important to realize the limits to your control, and not to blame yourself unjustly. But responsible people take the credit for what they have done well, and they assume ownership of mistakes they have made. When you find yourself blaming your son or your husband or your neighbor for a distressful situation you have gotten yourself into, say, "I made the decisions. I am responsible for the consequences. It's not his (or her) fault." Remember the difference between blaming and taking responsibility: the first accomplishes little but creating more anger and resentment, while the second can be constructive and appropriate.

8. Shoulds

If you hear yourself saying, "I should," "You must," or "We ought" a lot of the time, you are putting yourself and others in iron cages. "I should" implies that you have no choice. You are making rigid rules about how people *should* behave. Here is the key to unlocking the cage: *be flexible.* Recognize that you have choices about how to act. Let other people have free agency to make choices based on their values, not yours. If you have raised children, you know that each one came into the world with a different personality. You could discipline one with a whispered suggestion, while another required many trials before learning correct behavior. Allowing people to be different sets you free to be yourself, to operate in a manner that fits you. You might have very good reasons not to act as you think you "should" all the time. Can you think of personal needs that sometimes compel you to act against your values? Those needs might deserve compromise or accomodation. The same is true for others, their needs, and their values. Resist iron-clad rules.

Step 5

The final step on the Spot and Stop Record is to make a list of things, people, or events that you enjoy thinking about.

Spend some time thinking of positive things in your life, little things and big things, things that make you feel happy. Write them down under Part B of the Spot and Stop Record.

Sometimes strange things make people happy. When my daughter, at age 18, experienced a serious depression, she wrote a list of things to think about when having negative thoughts. She showed me the list, and the first thing was "Geranium on my windowsill." I laughed, and asked, "Why?" The geranium on her windowsill hadn't had much care. It was mostly a long, dry-looking stem with a few leaves toward the tip. It did always seem to have a red flower blooming, however. Maybe my daughter felt like that geranium. Perhaps it made her feel better to see that even when things look pretty bleak, there is still hope. I don't know. She didn't know, either, she just liked it.

The point is that you can put anything on your list. My grandchildren are on my list. I can pull myself out of the doldrums in an instant thinking about them. Sure, I worry about them, too, but just picturing their faces and remembering their dear ways is uplifting. This afternoon I have a four- and a six-year-old coming over to play games for an hour. I will be tired when they leave, but I will be in the best of spirits.

You have your own unique memories and things that make you feel happier. Keep the record handy so you can write down happy things whenever you think of them. This list is your resource when you start thinking negatively. When you find yourself awfulizing, personalizing, putting yourself down, or remembering something sad from the past, look at your record and start thinking about an item on your list. Don't choose, just think about the first one your eyes fall upon. You have to work at this. Doing it for just one day won't accomplish a change.

Marta's Spot and Stop Record

Although Marta was not what you would call an unpleasant person, she had days of feeling down, and on those days she wasn't very good company. It usually started around mid-morning after she had cleaned the kitchen and started a load of laundry. "I kind of run out of gas around that time," she said, "and then I look around at dust in the corners, and at the walls that need painting, and I just feel so discouraged because I don't have energy or money to do anything about it." There was a clue in her statement. Do you see it? To find it herself, Marta began to keep a Spot and Stop Record.

Marta said, "I don't have energy or money to do anything about it." She was able to look at the statement and identify what she had been saying to herself all morning: *Filtering* out the strength and resources she did have, and *Overgeneralizing* the difficulty of her situation. She talked to herself like this: "I've got to get this kitchen clean before I run out of gas [*Shoulds*]. Oh my, I hope the utility bill doesn't come before my social security check gets here [*Catastrophizing*]. I'm getting really tired now. I can't do any more [*Polarized Thinking*]. I'm done for the day. It's always like this...I'm never able to take care of things the way I should [*Filtering*]. What's the use?" When Marta wrote those thoughts down, she was impressed by how totally negative they were. Self-fulfilling, too, since the thoughts made her feel worse. "But what can I say?" she asked. "That's all true."

After considerable thought, Marta was able to change her statement to "I'll do half the kitchen tasks now, and then I'll sit down and rest for 10 minutes. Then I'll start the laundry, and while that's going I can write a letter to my sister. I'll have some applesauce, too, and that will give me a lift. After that I'll do one other task, maybe get those cobwebs over the piano. Each day I'll divide things up like that. I don't have to clean the whole kitchen every day. After lunch I'm going for a walk to enjoy the fall weather, and then I'll have a short rest, and maybe read that new book I got at the library." Marta felt better when she wrote her truthful, accurate statements down. They made sense, and they were positive. Her plan recognized her limitations, and contained realistic goals. She stated to herself that she was going to nurture and take care of herself. Look at her Spot and Stop Record on the next page to see how she identified the negative thoughts (underlining key words), and created rational comebacks.

Marta also listed the things she loved thinking about and enjoying during her breaks. The list reminded her to find room for pleasure each day, and that her life extended far beyond tiresome daily tasks.

Spot and Stop in Your Daily Life

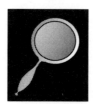

Now that you have your own repertoire of rational comebacks and pleasant topics to think about, you can practice the Spot and Stop procedure in your daily life.

Each and every time you hear yourself being a negative self-talker, yell "stop!" mentally or aloud.

"Stop!" is a powerful word. It brings to mind images of red stop signs, red traffic lights, a blue-clad policeman holding up his hand. It is the word you screamed in terror when your two-year-old ran into the street. It is the word that silenced a pair of quarreling brothers.

Practice saying "stop" now. Say it forcefully so the "s" hisses out strongly, and the "t" fires the "p" out of your mouth like a bullet. Say it six times, right out loud. That is the word you are going to say each time you catch yourself saying bad or unhappy things to yourself. Your motto from now on will be "Spot and Stop."

After you have forcefully "stopped!" your negative thought, challenge it by restating one of your rational comebacks. Then begin thinking about one of your preferred, happy subjects.

Most of the time your negative thoughts are brief flashes of a word or two, or even just a mental picture. You need some tricks for spotting these thoughts, and for stopping them quickly. Suppose you look in the mirror at withered breasts and wrinkled face, and find yourself saying, "Yuck!" or "Old hag." That is the time to spot the thought and stop it. You would look again at your breasts and say, "Stop! These are good breasts. They have been loved and caressed. They have nurtured a child and been a solace to a baby in pain. I love my breasts. They have served me well." This leads you naturally into pleasant memories of your child.

Spot and Stop Checklist

The way to be most effective in building new thought patterns is to record your progress. On the small Spot and Stop Checklist, you will now be able to keep track of your thought stopping without much bother. Just check the Spot column when you catch yourself in negative self-talk. Then check the Stop column to show you corrected your thinking, either by switching to some happy thoughts or by restructuring the old thought. Check the Feeling column to indicate that you have a new feeling. Just put G for good or

Spot and Stop Record
Marta's

Date: <u>June 1</u>

Part A

Spot	Stop	Rational Comebacks
(Negative Self-Talk)	(Negative Thought Patterns)	(Healthy, Accurate Self-Talk)
I don't have energy to do anything about all the cleaning needed.	Filtering strength I do have; overgeneralizing	I have energy to do half the tasks now, and half after I rest.
I've got to get this kitchen clean before I run out of gas.	Shoulds Polarized Thinking	Sometimes I'm too tired to clean. That's OK, I can do some each day.
I hope the utility bill doesn't come before my social security check gets here.	Catastrophizing	It hasn't happened yet. There are better things to think about now.
I'm never able to take care of things the way I should.	Filtering Shoulds	I took wonderful care of my children. I choose where to invest my energy.

Part B

My list of things, people, or events I enjoy: Taking an autumn walk. Reading a good book.

Having the grandchildren visit. Homemade applesauce.

Songs my mother used to play on the piano.

B for bad in that column. Most likely you will have all G's. If you have some B's showing up, you need to work a little harder at the stopping process. If the negative thoughts are not fully stopped, you will have bad feelings. Seeing mostly G's on your chart lets you know you are successful in changing your self-talk. If you can discipline yourself to keep this checklist for four weeks, you can be confident the new way of thinking will stick. Return to the list whenever you feel yourself slipping into old ways.

Marta used the checklist along with her Spot and Stop Record once she realized how negative her thinking had become. She enjoyed the feeling of actively taking charge and doing something to improve her mental state. At first she filled up one whole verticle column in a day and a half. As time went on and she became better at spotting and stopping, she noticed that she had fewer times each day to record negative thoughts. By the end of 36 days, positive self-talk had become as automatic as the negative self-talk used to be. Marta felt better, happier, and she had more energy. She was enjoying life. She smiled often.

Spot and Stop Checklist

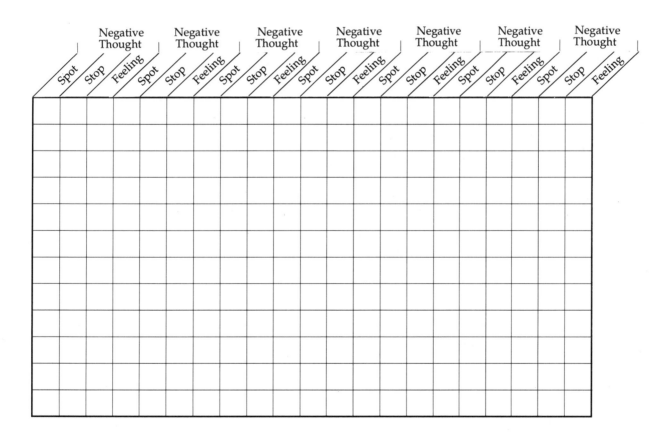

The Value of Positive Self-Talk

If you believe in life after death, you probably remember that scriptures tell us that our bodies will be restored in their best condition, even to every hair being accounted for. That means that you go into the next life with the same mind and all that you have learned in this lifetime. Do you want to have exactly the same thought patterns and personality that you have had in this life? Most people answer that question by saying, "Why, no! I want to be a happy, cheerful person. I don't want to feel anxious or angry or fearful. I want to have a good time over there and have other people enjoy being around me." Very few believe they are perfect just the way they are.

This realization, and this belief, are good motivators to work on becoming the happiest, pleasantest person you can possibly be. If you don't believe in life "beyond," you can still make your present life a lot better by becoming the happiest, pleasantest person you can possibly be.

The way to do this is to develop positive thinking. Norman Vincent Peale knew this back in 1950 when he first wrote *The Power of Positive Thinking*, which he later revised. James Allen knew it 90 years ago when he wrote *As a Man Thinketh*. Allen said, "A man is literally *what he thinks*, his character being the complete sum of all his thoughts." Allen learned it from studying the teachings of Jesus Christ. Even before the birth of Christ there were Greek philosophers who observed that morose thoughts produced morose people. The fact that so many have observed this and have written about it means that it is a very common failing to indulge in negative self-talk. It is worth time and energy to overcome it. You can do it.

Learning To Like Your Changing Self

Few people at age 70 look just as they did at 20; those who do have probably had a little surgical assistance. Your youth, and mine, were influenced by Hollywood glamour. People were supposed to look smooth-skinned, sexy, and gorgeous all the days of their lives. Old came to mean ugly. What a shame. That slick beauty was so shallow, but the media did a good job of making us think a wrinkle or a gray hair was a sign of social death. Have you seen "Driving Miss Daisy" with Jessica Tandy? Tandy's beauty is deeper than the thickness of her skin. And what about Kathryn Hepburn and Henry Fonda in "On Golden Pond"? Aren't they beautiful?

Like a lot of mothers, I used to tell my daughter, "Beauty is only skin deep" (her brother would say, "Yeah, but ugly goes clear to the bone"). The superficial vision of youth matches its flawless skin and trim figure. Years of experiencing success and failure, happiness and grief, make people beautiful in a better way than any Hollywood starlet could ever be. Do you believe that? Or do you only believe it in principle? When you look at how you've changed, do you resent the loss of superficial prettiness? Of course you do, sometimes.

Throughout this book you've been thinking about the question "Who am I?" Turn back the pages to your Living Systems Inventory, *Myself*, in Chapter 2 and see what you wrote about your assets and liabilities. What did you say about your physical appearance? Do those assets and liabilities still stand after you have been through the Spot and Stop process? Maybe you feel differently about some things now. Take time to revise your inventory. It will be interesting for you to see how much change there may be. Keeping your inventory current helps you to cement what you have learned.

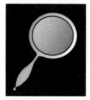 Chances are there are many assets you forgot to list on your original inventory. Now is the time to add to that list, dredging up your accomplishments throughout your life. The phrases below can help you remember a few more things you've done, learned, and accomplished. If there's no room on your inventory, write your new assets here.

I am
I made
I loved
I gave
I helped
I taught
I learned

When you have added at least five more assets to your list, review the entire list and select half a dozen that you feel especially good about. Print or type these assets on 3 by 5 cards, one asset to a card. Place one in your purse, one on a mirror, another on the refrigerator, and the rest in other places where you will see them every day. Whenever you feel down, or find yourself hating the changes in your body, go to one of these cards and spend five minutes thinking about the wonderful asset that came from the person who lives inside your body. When you are brushing your teeth, focus on the asset stuck to your mirror. You have that asset. You never lose assets. Even if negativity has taken over, the assets are still in there someplace, and thinking about them will bring them out.

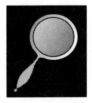 You probably have a collection of snapshots and studio pictures of your family. Dig them out of the shoe boxes and old albums, and take an afternoon to enjoy them. Do you have some of yourself as a child? As a teen? What about wedding pictures? And, of course, pictures of that first baby. Babies change so quickly into children, don't they? And the teen years! You would hardly know it was the same person. Seems like there are three or four major changes. The first comes at age six when you lose a tooth, get a haircut, and go to school. The next when you turn 13, and get braces on your teeth and maybe a few pimples on your face. Now who is this sophisticated young 20-year-old? Can that be you? Changes after that are gradual, but there comes a time — somewhere between 40 and 50 — when your face seems to be differently shaped, and your middle is a little thicker. The lines in your face are becoming noticeable, and in another decade or two they will be creases. Your hair turns, and for some it falls out. These changes are natural

events, just like losing your tooth at age six, or getting braces at 13. Who's at home inside? Isn't it the same person as the one without the tooth, or the one in the wedding picture?

I have heard many women say, and I have said it myself, that it is a great shock to get out of the shower and see a body that does not at all match the young girl who lives inside. Men don't talk about it as much, but that doesn't mean they don't feel it. One time I was sharing a shower with my daughter and granddaughter on a camping trip and Julia, age three, said, "Grammy has a wrinkled bottom." That kind of thing is a little hard on the ego, but wrinkles or not, the person who lives inside is still the same. You are now, and always will be, the person who lives inside your body. The body takes a lot of hard knocks in a lifetime, but the "me, myself, and I" remains. In the years after 50, self-acceptance depends upon knowing your inside person.

This reminds me of my husband's favorite chair. It is an old brown recliner pretending to look like leather. The footrest sags to one side a bit as a result of children sitting there. There are holes in the arms which have been patched with liquid vinyl. It doesn't match anything else in the room, and is really too large, for the room is rather small. Nevertheless, it has personality. It sits in benevolent honor, knowing it will never be displaced. My husband loves that chair. He is quite tall, and the chair fits him. I think his feelings for the chair and for me are somewhat the same. No matter how saggy or crooked we get, he will still love us. New chairs are pretty to look at, but old chairs are comfortable to know.

Gina

I'd like to tell you about Gina. I've known Gina for 30 years. We haven't always lived in the same town, but we've never lost touch. We did live near each other when our children were growing up, and I always admired the way Gina managed her large family. She was then a pretty young woman, bright and interesting. As in all families, some of her children had trouble making it through adolescence. One son became an alcoholic; his sister left home at 17 because she didn't want her parents to know she was pregnant. All of this took a toll on Gina. The lines around her mouth showed her grief. Then Gina found a lump in her breast. A biopsy showed cancer cells, and in those days they didn't do lumpectomies, they simply took the whole breast, along with lymph nodes and anything else that happened to be in the way. So at 40 she had only one breast. Throughout all of these trials Gina maintained concern for other people. Her grief about her daughter led her to become a volunteer at a pregnancy center where she could counsel young girls who faced the same fearful decisions her daughter had faced.

She attended Alanon to learn how to handle her son's alcoholism and be a support to the rest of the family. She used her tragedies as learning experiences in the hope that she could help her other children avoid these pitfalls. Gina had grit and determination. She was a good friend. She never allowed her own problems to interfere with compassionate interest in the concerns of her friends, or in the affairs of church and community. At 45 she celebrated the "five-mile mark," and believed herself to be free of cancer. She didn't like the mutilation of her body. The ugly scars where her breast used to be were repugnant. She never looked in the mirror until she was fully dressed. She believed she was no longer sexually appealing. She turned away from her husband, Rudy, in the night, unable to stand his hand upon the barren flesh. Rudy insisted he did not feel repulsed, but Gina couldn't believe him, at least not for a long time. Cosmetic surgery had never been suggested, and neither Gina nor Rudy thought of it. After a while, Gina did adjust; she accepted Rudy's love, although she never did feel quite the same about herself.

At 51 the cancer came back, requiring extensive surgery to remove tumors from her neck and face. During surgery, bone was removed from her face and a muscle was taken out of her neck, leaving Gina with a caved in and scarred face and neck. All that was left to remind us of the pretty face were her huge green eyes, framed with long, dark lashes. Gina felt violated and defiled. The experience had been dehumanizing, at best, and completely demoralizing. Gina lost track of who she was and why she was here. To Rudy, and to her friends, Gina was still Gina. Her "me, myself, and I" had not changed. She was still the warm, loving person we had always known. She was beautiful.

Gina was understandably depressed. She stayed depressed until her 60th birthday. Rudy knew he had to give Gina back her "self." He spent a lot of time on the phone with the children, trying to figure out something to do for Gina's birthday that would restore her sense of who she really was. Shelley, the daughter who had run away from home, had an idea.

"We could do a 'This is Your Life' kind of thing, Dad," she said.

"Well…" Rudy hesitated. "Isn't it kind of corny?"

"Yeah, it is," Shelley agreed, "but wouldn't it do what we want? I mean, wouldn't it show her all the wonderful things she is, whether she's scarred or not?"

Rudy thought about it. "I guess it might do that. OK…you check with Mike and Bob, and I'll talk to Denise and Karen."

"It's a deal," Shelly said.

Rudy did all of his calling from the office so Gina wouldn't know what they were cooking up. Actually, Gina was having some pretty serious thoughts about not being available on her birthday. "I don't want everyone looking at me," she thought. "They'll think they have to do something, and all I want to do is hide. I could say I was going to see my sister, and then I could really just go to a motel for a couple of days. I've never been deceitful before, but I can't stand having them feel sorry for me. I don't want the grandchildren to think they have to kiss this Frankenstein face."

As it turned out, Rudy had a feeling Gina would try to weasel out of her birthday, so they planned the celebration for the week before. When Gina said she might go to her sister's on her birthday, Rudy just smiled and said, "Fine. It'll do you good to get away."

On the day of the party, Gina and Rudy went to church, sitting at the back, as always. Gina always hoped no one would notice her. Of course, that didn't work because everyone loved Gina and wanted to talk to her.

Can't they see how embarrassed I am? thought Gina.

After church, Rudy said, "Honey, could we stop by Mike's on the way home? He has a special wrench that he thinks will fit on that furnace valve I haven't been able to fix."

Gina reluctantly agreed. "Oh well," she thought, "I'll get to see the baby, and he's too little to know I'm a freak."

When they parked at Mike's house, their son came out to the car to greet them. "Mom," he said, helping her out of the car, "you've got to see what little Rudy can do. He's rolling over all by himself." Gina's heart warmed at the thought of her grandchild, and she went quickly into the house, forgetting for a moment her embarrassment. Mike opened the door, and Gina stepped in. First she saw the big red banner that read, "Happy Birthday, Mom!" and then she heard, "Surprise…surprise," and was instantly enveloped in loving arms of all sizes. Tears flowed, and laughter followed. Gina was led to the seat of honor, and her life was presented before her. The grandchildren all had a part to play, of course, and the baby lay in Gina's arms, never knowing that his grandma thought she was ugly.

In this presentation, Gina's assets were made clear. The love her family had for her was too evident to be disbelieved. The ultimate offering was a large book containing pages contributed by family members and dozens of friends. Each person had prepared a page showing how important Gina had been in their lives. It was a unique way to let Gina see that she was still the same wonderful person she had always been. It was a door opening for Gina, the beginning of losing her self-consciousness and accepting herself in a changing body.

That's a dramatic way to get in touch with your inside self, and it may not happen to you in just that way. Of course, you could do it for someone else, I suppose. But you can do it for yourself, too. You might even want to write a story about yourself.

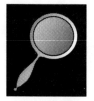 If you choose to write your own story, refer to your Complete Living Systems Inventory from Chapter 2. Use both the assets and liabilities columns, and be both honest and kind. In writing your story, you will see that there have been mistakes, sorrows, and tragedies, but you will also see that you are a strong and special person to have survived it all. You can see how your assets helped you in the hard times, and how they can help you now. You may find that you have more going for you than you realized. You aren't just one of "the aging," you are a person who has *had* an interesting life, one who has learned a lot. After my mother's death, I found a packet of letters with a note on top. It said, "For my girls, so they will know I had a life, too." They were letters from friends she was with when she was a Red Cross nurse back in the 1918 flu epidemic. My sister and I were touched that she lived this life of which we knew very little, and we were sad that we only learned of it after her death. She was a person. She wasn't only "mother." Accepting your own person, even though the package changes, puts you in a position of being in charge of your present and future life. Buy a spiral notebook and start writing.

By now you have had a pretty good look in the mirror. You probably have more understanding of things you already knew, and I hope you have some new insights, too. In the next chapter, you will build on these insights to help you become a stronger communicator and decision maker. You are going to take charge of your life. These skills will help you continue to make your life your own.

References

Allen, J. (1976) *As a Man Thinketh*. New York: Grosset & Dunlop.

Beck, A. (1979) *Cognitive Therapy and Emotional Disorders*. New York: New American Library.

Ellis, A. (1971) *Growth Through Reason*. Palo Alto, CA: Science and Behavior Books.

McKay, M., M. Davis, and P. Fanning (1981) *Thoughts and Feelings: The Art of Cognitive Stress Intervention*. Oakland, CA: New Harbinger Publications.

Peale, N.V. (1952) *The Power of Positive Thinking*. New York: Prentice-Hall, Inc.

4

Taking Charge

You have solved millions of problems in your life. When you were young, your parents and perhaps older siblings solved some of your problems for you. If you married, you probably found that problems and solutions had to be considered by your companion before they could be finalized. Sometimes marriages fall apart because one person insists on making all the decisions, thereby robbing a mate of a fundamental right. Sometimes a marriage is troubled because no one can be decisive, and problems are solved by default. How has it been in your life? Do you have a systematic way of examining and solving problems, or do you tend to wait until "fate" takes control? Are there instances where you wish you had formulated a clearer plan of action, but didn't, or couldn't? Whatever your habits in the past, now is a good time to become more organized in your approach to problems. Doing so will help you find those perfect solutions only you can know about.

This chapter has two parts: the first is about problem solving, and the second is about communication skills. You may be surprised to find that clear communication alone can solve many problems. While you've been communicating and solving problems all your life, you may not always have been satisfied with the way things have worked out. Now is your chance to master approaches that will help you decide what you want, and communicate well enough to get it.

Solving Problems

The key to solving most problems is to get as well organized a view of the situation as possible. Organization helps you see things objectively, consider them from many perspectives, and evaluate your options methodically. It doesn't mean losing your personal, emotional perspectives, which is an important consideration in any problem-solving process. It does mean leaving the feeling of being overwhelmed behind.

The first step in problem solving is identifying the true problem. It's easy to become overwhelmed by large issues, especially when they have many different facets or call up strong emotions. Thinking about a spouse's death, for instance, can be numbing. But focusing those thoughts on one issue at a time can make the situation more manageable. You might think first about what you'd do about your living situation; that presents a problem and a decision in itself. Once that issue is resolved, you can turn your thoughts to finances, or pets, or whatever problem you've identified as of secondary importance. The trick is to look at each problem separately.

Sometimes the real problem is not what it appears to be. In 1971 two researchers, Thomas D'Zurilla and Marvin Goldried, turned their scholarly attention to general problem solving and concluded that the real problems are *failures to find effective responses*. In other words, it is not the situation itself that is problematic — say, the fact that your spouse chews breakfast with his mouth open, driving you crazy — but the fact that your response — yelling, or pouting, or tearing your hair out — is ineffective, even self-destructive. If you realized that the true problem was your ineffective response, and not your spouse's manners, you could begin to solve the problem. Possible solutions would be more constructive responses on your part: discussing the issue politely with your spouse, choosing to be in a different part of the house while he ate, whatever. The important thing to remember is that you need to identify the part of the problem you can do something about. You want to eliminate the problem by finding an effective response.

There are four steps to the following problem-solving process. It is modeled on a problem-solving process devised by D'Zurilla and Goldried, and can help you address any problem methodically, rationally, and productively.

Four Steps to Problem-Solving

1. Write down the problem you face.

If you are confronting a large problem with many related issues, start by stating the big problem, and then listing everything else that comes to mind. If you don't know which is the main problem, list them all. Don't filter or prioritize anything yet — just get it all down.

For instance, Willa had been worrying about her living situation ever since her husband passed away. The children were pressuring her to sell the house, but the prospect terrified her. Where would she go? Would she be cut off from her memories and her friends and family? This is what Willa wrote:

Big Problem: Should I sell my house?

Related Problems: Will the children still visit me?
                    Can I afford to live anywhere as nice as this?
                    What if I stay and become unable to keep this place up?
                    Will I be saying I can't do the work I once did?

> Where will I go? Retirement center? Apartment? Not with the children — I couldn't do that again.
> Cleaning the house out will be hard. Leaving it and all its memories will be heart-rendering.
> Would I see my friends again if I left?

2. Pick the number one problem.

This is your chance to make sense of your problem list, creating a rational order of attack. Often, the number one problem will be one aspect of the big problem. Problems that are important to one person may not be so important to another. If money is not a problem, then the decision about whether to move after a mate's death is lower on the scale. A problem of higher priority might be legal matters pertaining to the estate. Only you can know how important a problem is. One way to think of it is in terms of time. That is, how soon does this problem need to be solved?

It's best to focus on only one problem at a time as you go through this process. You will come back to the next priority decision on the list once you have a clearer picture of how you'll respond to this more important issue.

For Willa, the question of where she would go was the heart of the issue. She'd want to come back to examine the other issues later, but finding an appealing alternative to her house was the real source of anxiety. The ideal solution would take into account some other problems as well, such as finances and family visits.

3. Brainstorm solutions to the number one problem.

Imagine every possible solution to the number one problem. Don't decide yet which ones might or might not work. Let your creative mind go to work without any filtering or blocking from your practical side. Write these solutions down.

For example, Willa wrote:

> Retirement center
> Apartment
> Move in with the kids

4. Evaluate likely solutions on the Consequences Chart.

The Consequences Chart on the next page can help you analyze possible solutions to your problem. It offers a methodical way of looking at present and future consequences of any particular decision. You may want to make several blank copies of the chart before you write in it so you can use it for further problem solving.

a. Pick what seems to be the number one solution. If you can't decide easily, pick any of the possible solutions — you'll have a chance to come back to the others later. Write this option at the top of your consequences chart.

For Willa, this was the retirement center. She didn't know much about it, but the kids mentioned it so often that it was the first thing that came to her mind.

Consequences Chart

Number one problem: _____

Possible solution: _____

Myself	Overall Quality of Life	Financial	Emotional Well-Being	Physical Health	Spiritual Life	Intellectual Development	Goal Achievement	Relationships	5 Years From Now	10 Years From Now	20 Years From Now		

+ = mostly good consequences

- = mostly bad consequences

0 = neutral

b. Consider the probable outcome of that solution in various areas of your life. You'll see categories written across the top of the Consequences Chart, such as emotional well-being, finances, and spiritual life. These are concerns many people have; you probably have a few specific ones of your own. Add those concerns in the blank spaces at the top right of the chart.

Now think about the probable outcome of the number one solution in each of your areas of concerns. If the outcome is mostly positive in that area, it gets a plus. If the outcome is mostly negative, it gets a minus. If you just can't decide or it doesn't matter, it gets a zero for neutral. In some cases, it can help to list all the possible outcomes on both sides, positive and negative, and count them to see which wins.

List your pluses, minuses, and zeroes in the first row, across from Myself, under the heading for each particular concern.

You'll see how Willa completed her chart and what her reasoning was, on the next page.

c. Consider who else is likely to be affected by the solution.

List every relevant person you can think of on the lines under Myself. Then, using the categories across the top, ask yourself how each person will be affected immediately, in five years, in 10 years, and in 20 years. Use pluses and minuses as you did above, and zeros if the category isn't relevant for that person.

In writing names down, you may realize that certain people have a right to a say in your decision. Depending on the situation, it is fair to decide that someone else should decide on a particular issue. It is also fair to solicit input, and still decide for yourself.

d. Count your pluses and minuses.

The best way to do this is to add the pluses and subtract the minuses. Write the total in the bottom row. It might be clear from glancing at the chart that you have a majority of pluses or of minuses. But a number lets you compare this solution to other solutions on your brainstorming list — solutions you can analyze in the same way, one at a time.

If you are thorough in examining every solution in the various categories, your answer should come more clearly into focus. Which has the most pluses? Which have the most important pluses? Which consequences can you envision as working best? As you can see, it is still important to bring subjective feelings into consideration, even after you've used numbers. The Consequences Chart helps you explore even these feelings in a methodical way. You may find it helpful to see how Willa approached her chart.

Willa's Chart

After completing steps 1 though 3, Willa realized that her number one problem was what to do about her living situation. The number one solution was moving to a retirement center — at least that was what came to her mind first. In the categories below, you'll see how Willa methodically examined each angle of that potential solution.

Willa's Consequences Chart

Number one problem: <u>Where would I go?</u>

Possible solution: <u>Retirement Center</u>

Willa's Chart	Overall Quality of Life	Financial	Emotional Well-Being	Physical Health	Spiritual Life	Intellectual Development	Goal Achievement	Relationships	5 Years From Now	10 Years From Now	20 Years From Now					
Myself	0	0	+	+	+	+	- + +	+ -	+ -	+	0					
Spouse	+	0	+	0	+	+	+	+	+	+	+					
Daughter	+	+ -	+	0	0	+	0	+	+	+	0					
Son-in-law	+	-	+	0	0	0	0	+	-	-	-					
Sister	+	0	+	0	+	+	+	+	+	+	0					
Brother	+	0	+	0	+	+	+	+	+	+	0					
Parent	0	0	+	0	+	+	+	+	0	0	0					
Neighbor	-	0	-	0	-	+	+	-	0	0	0					
Friends	+	0	+	0	+	+	0	+	0	0	0					
Total	+6	-1	+7	+1	+5	+8	+7	+6	+3	+4	+0					

+ = mostly good consequences
- = mostly bad consequences
0 = neutral

Overall Quality of Life

In the first column, Willa evaluated how the decision to move into a retirement center would affect her own life. Willa believed that the overall quality of her life would be positively affected because she would be relieved of lawn care, her apartment would be cleaned once a week, attractive meals would be served in the dining room, and she could use her energies for writing her family's history...something she had long wanted to do. Willa placed a "+" in that column.

Financial Security

Next, she considered financial security. Although the retirement home seemed expensive, she had to consider the fact that she would no longer be paying water or utility bills. She also would not be paying for food, except snacks, because these things were all included in the monthly fee. When she added up the monthly expenses involved in owning her own home, they were about equal to the retirement center fee. While it did not increase financial security, neither would it be jeopardized. Willa put a neutral "O" in that column.

Emotional Well-Being

There was no question in Willa's mind that living in the retirement center would be beneficial to her emotional well-being. For the past year she had felt increasingly uneasy, and at times very frightened, alone at night in her house. She loved her home, but it was an old house in an old neighborhood, and there had been an increase in crime in that area. In fact, on two occasions obscenities had been spray-painted on her fence. The couple two doors down had been burglarized the previous summer, and the woman across the street was mugged only last week when she came home from an evening meeting. At night, Willa slept restlessly, waking at every creak in the old house, every rustle of the leaves outside her bedroom window. There would be sadness, of course, at leaving the home she had shared with her husband and children, but it would be uplifting, too, to make a new nest for a new life. Plus on that one, she thought.

Physical Health

"I don't know that a change like this will have much affect on my physical health," Willa told her neighbor. "I guess I won't be as much at risk for accidents, you know...I won't be climbing ladders or trying to lift heavy things, so I guess it's a plus in that way." She also realized that she would be closer to medical help, and there was always someone there to call in an emergency. "Yes, it's a bigger plus than I thought," said Willa, marking her chart.

Spiritual Life

As Willa contemplated her spiritual life, both inner (in terms of beliefs) and outer (in terms of church-going activities), she had several things to consider. Were there likely to be people there who shared her values? Would she be able to attend her church on

Sundays? What about other meetings she enjoyed? She decided to investigate where she didn't have enough information.

"Let's see," she said to herself, "I can always get a ride with someone from the church, and anyway, they said their van makes the rounds to all the churches on Sunday morning." Willa took time to make phone calls so that she would be sure of transportation. Willa still drove, but her eyesight was not as good as it once was, and she preferred not to take the risk unless absolutely necessary. The next thing Willa did was to arrange to have lunch at the retirement center several times. Each time, she sat at a different table and thus obtained a fair sampling of the personalities and interests of the residents. She found two people from her church whom she had gotten to know very well. Finally, she was sure that from a spiritual point of view, it would be a good move. A "+" in that column.

Intellectual Development

The move was a plus for intellectual development because Willa would be free to pursue new interests. The center offered a book discussion group she might be able to join. She would also be encountering new people, which offered the chance for conversation and discovery.

Goal Achievement

Willa had long wanted to write a family history, but hadn't yet found the time. Moving would involve more time, and that was a minus since it would put the project off longer. But she might also find things in cleaning and packing that would help her write the story. And, of course, cleaning out the house was an important task. One minus and two pluses, Willa decided.

Relationships

Willa tried hard to find some liability with regard to relationships with her family and friends. She didn't want to jeopardize anything there, especially with the one son-in-law who so often disapproved of things she did. The only flaw she could find was that there would be no place for a whole family to sleep when they came to visit. That was both good and bad. She wanted her children to come as often as they could, and she loved having them. On the other hand, the physical work of providing three meals, snacks, and coping with the inevitable disorder that comes with children, was very taxing. Willa called one of the women she had met at lunch, and asked her opinion.

"I was worried about that, too," said Nancy, "but it has worked out just fine. They stay in a motel, and I pay for them to have meals with me here. It's really no more than I used to spend on food for them at home. In fact, it's more of a vacation for them because they can go back to the motel and let the kids swim, and they don't have to worry about me getting worn out. They always really enjoy the meals here, and I invite one grandchild each night to spend the night with me. You know, one child by himself is such a delight."

That sounded appealing to Willa, although she knew she couldn't count on everybody liking the arrangement. Still there were probably more pluses than minuses, so she compromised and put one of each.

Future Effects

Willa's next task was to consider the overall effects of her decision 5, 10, and 20 years in the future. This required a realistic appraisal of the state of her health, finances, and the limitations of the retirement center. The center she was considering did not have assisted living, so that would mean she could not stay there if she became unable to take care of herself. She knew that if she made some decisions now about these things, she would not have to worry about others making them for her. Her answers about the future had to be tentative, and she realized she would need new charts for other decisions to be made in the future.

Other People

Willa went through this same process again and again for each person listed on her chart. Notice that Willa included her husband, even though he is deceased. He is very much alive in Willa's mind, and therefore her questions concern her feelings about him and what he would think.

Final Evaluation

Adding up the pluses and subtracting the minuses told Willa that the pluses were in the majority. If they had come out about equal, she would have needed to reevaluate. She might want to take another look at the "O's" that follow her daughter's name. One thing she could do would be to talk with her daughter and see if her perceptions are correct. There also seems to be ambiguity about the impact of her decision on a neighbor who has depended on Willa for many years. A chat with the neighbor about her concerns might help to clarify things for Willa, and would also give an opportunity for the neighbor to feel included in Willa's new life. In Willa's case, it was easy to make the decision and carry it out without fearful doubts.

In every chapter from now on, you will be solving problems and making decisions. In fact, in the next chapter, you are going to make decisions related to health and prevention of problems. It is best to look at this project as a long-term affair. Take your time, and be thorough. If you do this, the coming years are going to be easier and more pleasant, no matter what may happen.

Successful decision making involves others. Willa needed to talk with her daughter and her neighbor. She needed to have good communication skills in order to be clear about her needs, and to be able to hear and understand what her daughter and her neighbor had to say.

Communication Skills

One of the privileges I have in life is to teach music to my grandchildren. I used to teach other children as well, but now I think the grandchildren are enough. My four-year-old granddaughter's piano lesson is understandably quite short. When she's had enough, she simply says, "That's all," and climbs down from the bench. Her statement is beautifully clear and direct, and her behavior reinforces her statement. The older children, through the process of going to school and observing the communication patterns of many adults and children, have learned to communicate in a different way. When they think the lesson has gone on long enough, they don't say, "That's all." They slump, they fidget, or they resort to silliness, and they start making lots of mistakes. I know what they're telling me, but if I ask, "Had about enough for today?" they usually say, "No, I'm just restless." Why do they do this?

First, they've learned in school that they have no power. The teacher has the power. When they get tired and bored in school, they are not allowed to say, "That's all," and go out for play. The teacher decides when they can have a break. You learned that, too, didn't you? And that kind of learning sticks with you. I played violin in symphony orchestras for 30 years. Everyone agrees that it is damaging to the player's body to play longer than 30 or 40 minutes without a break. For the past 10 years, there has been great interest in preventing injuries in musicians. That is, doctors and musicians are interested in this, but conductors are not. An orchestra rehearsal customarily goes for an hour to an hour and a half before taking a 10-minute break, and then they rehearse for that long again. Do these intelligent adult players ever say, "That's all," and walk off for a break? Never. You only do that if your bladder is so full that you are in imminent danger of flooding the place. And you think three times about that. If you visit a rehearsal of your local community symphony, you will see the players grimacing with pain as they massage a shoulder or turn their heads back and forth trying to relieve the muscle spasms. Think about situations you have been in where you were tired, bored, and badly in need of a break. Did you say, "That's all"?

The second reason children, and adults, do not state their needs in clear terms is fear. Fear of giving offense, fear of not being liked, fear of being abused, fear of ridicule, or fear of losing someone or something. You may think of other fears. I noticed something interesting at the Older American Center, where a noon meal is provided for a small donation. The older and poorer the diner, the less likely he or she is to criticize the food. It brought tears to my eyes to realize that these gentle friends are afraid the good, warm food will be taken from them.

There is a way to state what you think and feel and need without offending or risking unpleasant consequences. No person has teacherly authority over you. You can say, "That's all," and it will be OK. Here's how to do it.

There are two parts to effective communication: giving a message, verbally and nonverbally, and receiving a message, or listening. Let's start with giving messages.

Speaking in "I" Statements

A clear, direct statement says how you see a situation, what you feel, and what you want. The trick to effective communication is to incorporate all these elements, beginning each statement with "I."

When you say "I think," "I feel," "I want," you rarely offend the listener. You also make it impossible for the listener to disagree. When, on the other hand, you begin with "you," the tendency is to sound accusatory. "You never listen to me" is different from "I feel unheard." Can you see why one statement invites defense and disagreement, and the other sympathy and concern?

Using "I" statements also helps you focus on just what you think, want, and feel. When you are clear yourself on these issues, it becomes much easier to communicate them clearly to other people.

Think of it as a rule: always use "I" statements when you want to communicate an opinion, desire, or accusation.

Carol

Carol's children think she ought to be in a nursing home because she gets confused about whether she took her medicine or not, and on occasion she has taken a double dose by mistake. Carol thought that she would get along fine if someone could remind her about the medicine and maybe check up on her each day. But she didn't know how to tell the children what she wanted. She was afraid they would be annoyed with her and feel she was a burden. This is what she said: "Nursing homes are fine, but I'm not sick…well, I mean, I do need this medicine, but I'm not really…you know, sick. Getting older isn't much fun…I mean, it's just hard to figure out what to do about things."

Do you get any sense at all about what Carol really thinks? Or what she wants to do? No wonder her children see her as confused.

If Carol had used "I" statements, she might have been more successful. "I feel capable of caring for myself, although I need reminders of certain regular things," she might have said. This would have helped Carol and her children focus on more appropriate solutions to Carol's difficulties. "I want help, but not full-time care" would have shown her children that Carol had a clear sense of her own interests and limitations. Without those statements, Carol came across as confused.

Of course, Carol was nervous about discussing this issue with her children. When you're flustered, it's hard to be truthful, tactful, and focused. That's why the best solution is often to plan such encounters in advance. Carol might well have come up with perfect "I" statements if she had sat down with pen and paper to think about what she really wanted, before the children came over to discuss it. Simply writing the words "I think…," "I want…," and "I feel…" can be wonderful focusing devices.

Scripting "I" Statements

You'll want to script your "I" statements in advance any time you have a part in an important decision, such as Carol's. It's also a good idea to plan "I" statements whenever you think a discussion may lead to conflict. When you sit down to plan your statements, you have two goals in mind: first, to find out exactly what you think, feel, and want; and second, to plan your exact wording of important statements to ensure maximal impact.

Dorothea

Dorothea knew she was facing a big blowup with her family if she resisted their demands that she move in with her oldest daughter. "I raised them up to be strong and independent," she said to her neighbor, "but sometimes I think I created monsters." The problem was that Dorothea, who was also strong and independent, could no longer see to give herself the insulin injections she needed. "They think that's a problem," she said, "but I don't." Dorothea decided to prepare for the "conference" by organizing her thoughts into "I think," "I feel," and "I want" statements. She began writing an objective statement of the problem. By the end, she was able to put her thoughts together into a clear and decisive "I" statement. This is what she wrote:

1. The Situation: The family is coming on Friday, and I already know they want me to live with Irena, and I already know I'm not going to do that.

2. What I think it's about: I think they are afraid, and want to protect me. But I also think that I am more capable than they realize.

3. How it makes me feel: I feel cornered and downtrodden by their domineering attitude. No, wait...I can say that better. I appreciate their concern, but I feel intimidated.

4. What I want: This one's easy: I want to be respected for what I can do, and I want to live independently. I know I can buy those syringes with the insulin already in them, and I know I can inject myself just by feel. Good heavens, I've been doing it for 25 years. I want a home health nurse to check my blood with the glucometer.

5. What I'll say: OK, this is what I'm going to say to that loveable bunch of independent kids: "I think we have two different views of this situation. You appear to be worried about my ability to take care of myself, and I appreciate that. I think that I can take care of myself quite well with a little help. I really feel intimidated right now with this pressure to give up my independence and move in with Irena. Goodness knows, I love Irena and Bill and the kids with all my heart, but I'm not willing to make that move yet. This is what I want to do: I want to buy the prefilled insulin syringes and continue to give my own injections. After 25 years, I know by feel just how to do it. I also want to arrange for a home health nurse to come by and check my blood with the glucometer. I know I don't see well enough to do that. I hope that you can respect my wishes in this, as it is very important to me."

As it turned out, Dorothea got her way, and was able to live alone for several more years. The steps below can help you organize this process just as Dorothea did. Treat it as an exercise, if you like, writing your answers in and looking to Dorothea's statements as examples.

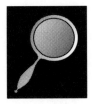 1. The Situation: Recall a recent situation in which you needed to express your opinion, your feelings, and your needs. Or, if you prefer, think about a situation that's coming up, or an old issue that is still unresolved.

2. Write down exactly what you *think* the situation is about. This is your chance to define the issue: you want to offer a *description* rather than an *opinion*.

I think:

3. Write down how you *feel* about the situation. What emotion does it trigger in you? What fears? What frustrations? What hopes?

I feel:

4. Write down what you *want* from the situation. Look inside yourself as you imagine different outcomes, and see what resolution would most satisfy you.

I want:

5. Now make up some complete *"I" statements* incorporating all three elements: "I think," "I feel," and "I want."

Being able to express your thoughts, feelings, and wants in a clear way is the first half of good communication.

Active Listening

The other component of clear communication is listening. You never offend people by really listening to what they say. Listening doesn't mean remaining silent while someone else talks. If you are going to be a good listener, you can't be busily making up something to say back, and you can't be judging what the other person is telling you. A good listener is focused on the other person, intent upon taking in what he or she thinks and feels and wants, whether that person is good at saying it or not.

The best way to listen effectively is to reflect back to the person what you think he or she said. That helps to make sure you did understand correctly — and it lets the other person know that his or her message is registering. Think of it as the rule of listening: *never offer your own response before you have confirmed that you understand the message being delivered.*

To confirm the message, simply ask the speaker if you got it right. Phrases like "What I hear you saying is…" and "It sounds like you think/feel/want…" will help you reflect the message back. The speaker will let you know if you missed the point. When he or she rephrases or repeats the message, reflect it back again. Only when the speaker looks relieved and says "That's it!" or "Yes, that's what I mean" can you proceed with your part of the conversation. You will both benefit from this rock-solid understanding of the speaker's message — and, if you're lucky, the listener will then take similar care to understand what you are saying.

It makes people feel good to be heard. If you pay careful attention to those who speak to you, and demonstrate this by reflecting exactly what you hear, you are already providing great comfort and support. People will feel comfortable sharing their problems with you. What's more, your responses to other people's questions and worries are more likely to be on-target when you understand things from their perspective.

A Conversation

Unfortunately, not everyone will listen as carefully as you do. It is therefore your job to make sure each person understands the other's point in a conversation. If you feel your point is not understood, even after careful "I" statement phrasing, ask the other person to reflect it back to you. To express "I feel that my point isn't being heard," you might say, "Can you tell me what you think I said?" If what the person says is not what you meant, express your point again using a new "I" statement. Keep this circuit going until you are able to say, "Yes, that's just what I mean." You'll be amazed at how much progress can be made in any situation merely by an understanding of the other's perspectives. A therapist I know mediated the following conversation, which illustrates how effective listening can be. Sometimes it's all it takes to solve a problem.

Daughter:	Whenever we speak, you talk to me about your new wife—what she's doing, wearing, thinking, planning. Sometimes you tell me a little about yourself, but you never ask about me, and what I'm up to. Don't you care?
Father:	*(reflecting/not yet responding/not becoming defensive at the "you" statement)* It sounds like you think I'm not interested in your life.
Daughter:	Well…(shaking her head) the problem is, I don't know if you're interested. You don't ask questions, so I can't tell what you think or even know about what's going on with me.
Father:	*(reflecting again, waiting for go-ahead)* So, you'd like it if I asked more questions about the details of your life?

Daughter:	Yes. That's what I want.
Father:	*(responding/careful to use "I" statement)* Well, I would like very much to know more about your life. But…I feel afraid that you'll think I'm prying. I want you to feel loved no matter what you do.
Daughter:	Prying? I would never feel that you were prying by asking me what I was doing—I *want* you to know. I guess I need to hear your interest to feel loved.
Father:	*(reflecting)* Are you saying that would be a sign that I love and care for you?
Daughter:	*(nods)*
Father:	*(given the green light to respond)* Why, that's wonderful news. Of course I love you and I care about you, and I feel sad that I haven't been showing that love in a way that you could see. But now I'm looking forward to asking all the questions I've been wanting to. Just — promise you'll let me know if I do start to pry?
Daughter:	I promise, Dad.
Father:	OK. So how is that new boss at work? She sounds like an ogre… *(they laugh)*

Strong communication skills will help you in every walk of life, from the most intimate to the most formal. Your relationship with family members can benefit, and so can your relationship with doctors and other professionals — something you'll be considering in more detail in coming chapters. Knowing how to speak clearly, and how to address problems clearly, won't make your problem go away. It's up to you to decide what you're saying, and what you're deciding after all. But isn't it worth a risk to know that your life is built around your own decisions? Far better to live your own mistakes, I say, than to live someone else's. Speak up and be heard.

References

D'Zurilla, T.J., and M.R. Goldried, (1971) "Problem Solving and Behavior Modifications." *Journal of Abnormal Psychology* 78: 107-126.

Lange A. J., and P. Jakubowski (1976) *Responsible Assertive Behavior*. Champaign, IL: Research Press.

McKay, M., M. Davis, and P. Fanning. (1988) *Messages, The Communication Skills Book*. Oakland, CA: New Harbinger Publications, Inc.

McKay, M., M. Davis, and P. Fanning. (1981) *Thoughts and Feelings, The Art of Cognitive Stress Intervention*. Oakland, CA: New Harbinger Publications.

5

Preserving Health

Thousands of books have been written about health — diet books, exercise books, books about preventive medicine and holistic health care, and so on. More will be written. You'd think it was some new and wonderful discovery. Actually, it is a *re*discovery, for it has been known through the ages that abusing the human machine will result in illness.

Desiderius Erasmus, Dutch humanist and editor of the first published edition of the New Testament, gave this advice in the 15th century:

> Avoid late and unseasonable studies for they murder Wit and are very prejudicial to Health. The Muses love the Morning, and that is a fit Time to Study. After you have din'd, either divert yourself at some Exercises, or take a Walk, and discourse merrily, and Study between whiles. As for Diet, eat only as much as shall be sufficient to preserve Health, and not as much or more than the Appetite may crave. Before Supper, take a little Walk, and do the same after Supper. A little before you go to sleep read something that is exquisite, and worth remembering; and contemplate upon it till you fall asleep: and when you awake in the Morning, call yourself to an Account for it.

Quite a while later, in 1916, Charles Wilkinson, a football coach, said, "People would be better off if they depended upon exercise rather than a drink for relaxation."

And finally, this statement by physician George W. Crane: "Any machine, whether the human body or an automobile, will obviously wear out sooner if it is overworked, mistreated, improperly lubricated, or fed chemicals that leave a residue of carbon around the valves! So treat your marvelous human machine far more carefully than a Rolls Royce!"

In the neighborhood where I live and work, there are many young people of middle- and high-school age. They appear to live on tacos, burgers, fries, and soft drinks. It is the cool thing to do. When I was in high school, the cool thing was to bring a brown-bag lunch, which usually contained a sandwich, carrot sticks, an apple, and a couple of cookies. It was standard fare; everyone's bag contained the same thing. The only use we made of the high school cafeteria was to have a place to sit, and to buy an ice cream after lunch. Ten years before that, in the same school, the "in" thing was to buy the cafeteria lunch. How was it when you were in school? What were the food habits of your peers?

Adolescent eating habits tend to become rather firmly entrenched. Chances are, you still like most of the same food you did when you were in high school. Sometimes these eating habits have bad effects on your health later in life.

Ralph, for example, grew up in a home where mom cooked with pure butter. She used butter to pan-fry meat. Butter was the choice for baking cookies and cakes. Cream went into sauces and gravies. There were always chocolate bonbons in pretty little dishes sitting around the house. Ralph liked these tasty foods, as who wouldn't? Unfortunately, Ralph's mother died at age 74 after several years in a vegetative state. The arteries to her brain were nearly closed, clogged with fatty deposits. When Ralph was 70, his doctor thought to check his cholesterol, low-density lipids, and high-density lipid levels. A few days later Ralph was informed that his cholesterol level was 280, and he was strongly encouraged to change his diet.

Sometimes, as you get older, you lose interest in food. It's too much trouble, perhaps, or it simply doesn't taste as good as it used to. Malnutrition is a contributing cause in the deaths of many people. This does not necessarily happen because of financial hardship — it happens to people of all income levels. Some of the reasons might be painful gums, or poorly fitted dentures, and even not having enough teeth in the right places. You may lose your appetite when you are ill, or if you are depressed. Fortunately, malnutrition is preventable, and so that is the first focus of your health improvement program.

Good Eating

The United States Department of Health and Human Services publishes a booklet called "Diet, Nutrition, and Cancer Prevention." This is a fine resource, which you can get from your local Cancer Society or by calling 1-800-4-CANCER. The dietary guidelines are appropriate, whether you are concerned about cancer or not. It is wise to note that the incidence of cancer is age-related, but some forms of cancer, such as colorectal cancer, are directly related to diet. In 1990 there were 145,000 cases of colorectal cancer in the United States. Twenty to 15 percent of cases occur in the rectum, the area most easily cured. Sixty to 63 percent are in reach of a sigmoidoscope. Obviously, early identification of these cancers increases the likelihood of cure. Of colorectal cancers that are found in the earliest stage, 95 percent can be cured with surgery. There is a hereditary factor, also, and if you have relatives who have had colorectal cancer, you would be well-advised to have yearly checkups. And, of course, to pay attention to your diet.

The government booklet states unequivocally that diets high in fiber, low in fat, and with plenty of fresh fruits, vegetables, and whole grains may reduce the risk of cancer. Beans and other legumes are also recommended. Dr. Stephen Axthelm, a surgeon at St. Mary's Regional Medical Center in Grand Junction, CO, confirms this, explaining that fiber keeps bile salts from irritating the lining cells of the colon. Another reason fiber is useful in preventing cancer is that it passes through the colon within 12 to 16 hours, as opposed to the slower 36- to 48-hour transit of low-fiber foods such as meat. Dr. Axthelm also points out that food in the cabbage family, such as broccoli and cauliflower, are thought to strengthen the immune system, thereby enabling the body to overcome cancers as they arise.

The cancer prevention diet has also been proven to lower blood cholesterol levels by as much as 25 percent or more when combined with an exercise program. Ralph, who consumed so much butter and cream as he was growing up, found that adherence to a diet such as the one described in the booklet brought his cholesterol down to 200 in about nine months. He also increased his exercise and used nutritional supplements to help his system correct the imbalance.

The dietary guidelines outlined here are for people of average health. If you have diabetes, or some other serious illness, the amounts of certain foods or the frequency of meals may need to be adjusted. If you are ill, you need to have an ongoing relationship with your primary care doctor. This book can be an aid, but it does not replace competent medical care. Here is what is recommended by the United States Department of Health and Human Services.

Dietary Guidelines

1. Eat a variety of foods.

One good rule is to have at least three different colors of food on your plate at every meal. For example, you might have a pasta or potato, a green vegetable, and one or more yellow/orange vegetables such as carrots, yams, or squash. Complete the meal with a whole grain bread or muffin, and for dessert, a baked apple. This goes a long way toward giving you the maximum amount of the 40 to 60 nutrients, but you may still need some vitamin or other food supplement.

2. Maintain ideal weight.

You won't find your ideal weight on a chart. Most people have had fluctuating weight over the years, and the weight that is best at age 60 is usually quite different from the weight you enjoyed at 25, even though you may have sustained the same height. Hundreds of factors affect the way your body metabolizes food, and those factors may change during childbearing, menopause, stress, illness, and certain drug treatments.

Your body will find the right weight if you eat the right foods when you are genuinely hungry, without worrying about calories or stringent diet programs. Your goal should be a state of good health, not thinness. The exception to this would be if you are seriously obese, or if you have diabetes or heart disease, in which case you need your doctor's help.

3. Avoid too much fat — all kinds of fat — and cholesterol.

The way to do this is to read labels on everything you buy. You want products that have less than five grams of fat per serving, and preferably less. Also, check to see what percentage of calories come from fat. If 100 percent of the calories come from fat, don't buy the product. Look for foods in which less than 25 percent of the calories come from fat.

Of course, you will want to avoid cholesterol, but don't be misled by labels that say "cholesterol free," because those products can still have a lot of fat. Only animal products contain cholesterol, but many other foods contain fat. Animal products include eggs, milk, cheese, and meat. An avocado is a vegetable that contains no cholesterol, but is high in fat. Beef and pork are heavily laden with both cholesterol *and* fat. Most vegetables are low in fat. Exceptions, besides avocados, are coconuts, nuts, seeds, and chocolate, which is derived from a vegetable. Sources for finding the fat and cholesterol contents of foods may be found at the end of this chapter in the nutrition chart. Remember, when you shop...look for the fat!

4. Eat foods that contain starch and fiber.

Remember when everyone thought starchy food would make you fat? Well, that's a myth that has been debunked. Potatoes, for example, are starchy, but contain no fat. A slice of bread has only one gram of fat. The only way potatoes and bread can make you fat is when they are laden with gravy, butter, or sugar-rich jams. The same is true of pasta. Fiber is found in fruits, vegetables, grains, and legumes — including potatoes, pasta, and bread. Meat is not a fiber food. There are wonderful recipes for meatless pasta. Stir-fried vegetables over rice are delicious and virtually fat free. When I say stir "fried," I'm not referring to the traditional method of using hot oil to fry the vegetables. You can use tomato juice, defatted chicken broth, fruit juice, or the liquid left from cooking beans. Eating the whole food is another way to get fiber — the skin of a baked potato, whole wheat breads and cereals, brown rice, and so forth.

5. Avoid sugar.

Try to use sweeteners that have nutritional value. Frozen juice concentrates, right out of the can, are very sweet. Bananas are good for sweetening drinks, muffins, and other baked goods. Honey is sweeter than sugar and has very small amounts of vitamins and minerals; sugar is purely empty of anything but calories. If you wish to replace sugar with honey in a recipe, reduce the amount of liquid by one-fourth cup for each cup of honey. Molasses is similar to honey in sweetness but has a stronger flavor. It does have the advantage of containing a small amount of calcium.

6. Avoid sodium.

The New Pritikin Program advises no salt at all. In truth, most vegetables and fruits contain some salt naturally, and a few, like celery, contain quite a bit. Seasoning with basil, oregano, parsley, thyme, and spices reduces the need for salt.

7. Avoid alcohol.

The benefits of small amounts of alcohol have been debated, but the liabilities seem to outweigh the benefits. Alcohol provides many "empty" calories — calories with no nutritional benefit at all — and depletes your system of valuable nutrients such as the B vitamins. There are better ways to relax. Try yoga, self-hypnosis, progressive relaxation, or just going for a leisurely walk. (You'll find more about healthful relaxation techniques in the next chapter.) Listening to your favorite music or talking to someone you love on the telephone will do more for you than alcohol.

8. Eliminate tobacco.

Just don't smoke, period. Smoking is a hard habit to break, but it can be done. If you need help overcoming your smoking habit, you might like to take a look at my book, *The Habit Control Workbook* (available by mail order, or from your book store). You could also go to a smoke-enders' clinic, listed in your local yellow pages.

Tobacco has no beneficial effects whatsoever, whether chewed or smoked. In concentrated form, nicotine is a highly toxic poison, and is a primary culprit in emphysema, cancer, and heart disease. When you smoke, everyone around you is at risk for these diseases.

9. Drink plenty of water.

Water serves to hydrate body tissues, and since your body is made up of water more than anything else, you can be sure that you need to respect the need for lots of water. Water serves to flush out toxins. Some doctors advise six to eight glasses a day, but don't specify what size glass. Others suggest drinking up to two quarts every day. I find it helpful to keep a glass of water by my work space, as well as by the bedside. I'm more apt to drink water if I don't have to go to the kitchen to get it.

Your body needs fuel. You can't expect it to ward off disease, heal broken bones, or keep you mentally alert if you don't give it what it needs. You know that you need vitamins and minerals in addition to protein, carbohydrates, and fiber. Vitamins, unlike carbohydrates, fats, and protein, are not broken down by the body into other substances for use in metabolism. Vitamins retain their original form in the body and are built into the body structure, where they become part of the machinery of the cells. The presence or absence of vitamins can mean the difference between illness and health. Vitamins need to be in small amounts and in the correct balance. You get vitamins from plant and animal foods or from supplements.

Theoretically, it should be possible to get all the vitamins you need just from plant foods, such as green leaves and stalks, root vegetables, fruits, seeds, beans, peas, kernels of wheat and corn, and sprouts. Realistically, there are factors which make this difficult to do. There are too many insecticides and fungicides in use, for one thing. These things affect the nutritional content of the plants, and they also affect your body's ability to absorb nutritional elements. There is also the problem, for some, of preparing, chewing, and digesting all the foods needed to maintain health. Nutritional supplementation, particularly for older people, is essential. Many doctors are not well trained in nutrition. Some have no training at all. You may have to seek advice from other sources, such as those described in the section on alternative health care in Chapter 7.

Grace

Grace's experience is fairly typical. She had always been a finicky eater. As a child she would only eat one thing, maybe mashed potatoes, and then after a few weeks of that she would eat only meat. Of course, she got over that. Her parents scolded and cajoled, finally giving up, and gradually she developed more normal eating behaviors. Even so, she wasn't much for vegetables.

At various times in her life — during the teen years and during pregnancy — Grace went through other phases of funny eating. For nearly a year she lived on potato chips dipped in cola drinks.

During pregnancy, all-day nausea pulled Grace right back to the mashed-potato-only days. Then there was the period when the only thing she desired was chow mein, the canned variety. Grace and Tim had chow mein every night for three months. Along about the fifth month, Grace felt better and resolved to get back to better eating habits. That's the way it went, all through the years. Pregnancy or illness meant funny eating.

After the last child left home, Grace experienced a big chocolate-craving period, which resulted in a 40-pound weight gain. She wasn't feeling well, either.

During the course of an annual physical exam, various lab tests were done. The doctor called Grace a week later. "I think you're in a little bit of trouble, Grace," he said. "Your cholesterol, LDL, and HDL are way out of control."

"Uh-oh," said Grace, "that means diet, doesn't it?"

The doctor then outlined for Grace a new plan of eating, similar to that described earlier in this chapter. He also recommended an exercise program.

"I'll send you some printed instructions," he said, "but I would like you to do some research on your own. I've found that the people who do the best at lowering their cholesterol do it on their own. Will you give it a try?"

Grace was more than willing. She followed the nine-step program in this book, and her cholesterol began a steady decline. After a time, she realized she was feeling better, with more energy, and that her clothes were getting a bit loose. Grace was motivated to learn and to try, and she improved the quality of her life.

Did You Know...
HDL, or High-Density Lipids, should be between 35 to 50?
LDL, or Low-Density Lipids, should never go above 100?
Cholesterol should be below 200?

The average cholesterol level for adults in the United States is about 215 to 220 mg/100 ml blood. That means that half the population is above that figure, and half below. If you look at the statistics on heart disease deaths, you will see that the cholesterol levels in heart patients who were studied ranged from 160 to 300. Therefore, if you keep your cholesterol at *or below* 160, your risk for heart disease is greatly reduced.

Three Steps to Health Improvement

These first steps to health improvement are related to things you put into your mouth. The blank record on the next page will help you do this in a systematic, organized way, for that is the best pathway to success. Before beginning, make several blank copies of the record — you'll be starting anew before long.

1. Record what you eat.

On the "Everything I Consume Record" on the next page, write down everything you put into your mouth for one week. Include *everything*: chewing gum, breath mints, cigarettes, drugs, drinks of any kind (including how much water you drink), and anything else not mentioned. Be honest. Chances are you are sincere in wanting to improve your health. Chances are you want to do everything you can to have a keen, clear mind so that you can make important decisions as you grow older. After all, you are still reading this book. Now all you have to do is act upon what you have read. You needn't make any changes the first week, because all you're going to do is record how things are now.

2. Analyze your record.

Are you surprised at what you see on your record? Do you eat more or less than you thought? How much variety is there? How much are you smoking? What, and how much, are you drinking? Are the foods high in fat? Consult the nutrition chart at the end of the chapter to see. Are the foods you chose nutritious? Draw a smiley face — or buy some smiley face stickers — by each food *low* in fat. Draw a big red X by each food *high* in fat. Now draw a red circle around the empty calorie, high-sugar foods like candy, sugary cereals, alcohol, and caffeine drinks. When you are through, you can see at a glance the proportion of undesirables to desirables. Now you have an idea about how drastic your change will need to be.

3. Plan appropriate changes.

It's time to make a decision. Study your record, and decide on one thing you will change this next week. Choose from the following list. These are imperative changes, but you should tackle only one at a time. If you try to make many changes all at once, you will upset your body too much. You don't want to become discouraged, so just one change, please.

Choose One:

1. *Stop smoking*. Do it cold turkey. Endure a week of agony, and get it over with. Every puff you take is worse than eating T-bone steak every night. Smoking will hasten your death. Research shows that those who successfully stop smoking do it on their own, and they do it cold turkey.
2. *Reduce alcohol intake*. If you drink to relax, there are better ways to do it, as you will see in the next chapter. More than one or two drinks a day severely shortens your life span. Even better would be to stop drinking all together.

Everything I Consume Record

Week Beginning: _____

Day 1:
Morning: _____

Midday: _____

Evening: _____

Day 2:
Morning: _____

Midday: _____

Evening: _____

Day 3:
Morning: _____

Midday: _____

Evening: _____

Day 4:
Morning: _____

Midday: _____

Evening: _____

Day 5:
Morning: _____

Midday: _____

Evening: _____

Day 6:
Morning: _____

Midday: _____

Evening: _____

Day 7:
Morning: _____

Midday: _____

Evening: _____

3. *Start drinking water.* Older people dehydrate easily, as you already know by your dry skin, dry eyes, and dry hair. Keep a big glass of water nearby — always, and drink from it often. Aim for one-and-a-half to two quarts a day.

4. *Drink fewer caffeinated and carbonated drinks.* Caffeine contributes to the development of osteoporosis, and has other deleterious effects. All carbonated drinks, because they contain carbonic acid, pull calcium from your bones. It would be ideal if you drank less than two or three of these a week.

5. *Add a raw vegetable to your noon and evening meals.* If you have difficulty chewing something as hard as a raw carrot, then have it lightly steamed, but avoid cooking for more than one to three minutes. The advantage to eating vegetables raw is that the vitamin and mineral content is not compromised.

6. *Add fresh fruit to your daily fare, preferably as snacks between meals.* The reason for not having fruit with meals is that fruit is digested faster than other foods. If you mingle fruit with other foods, it will be slowed in its journey while other foods are processed.

7. *Reduce sugar intake.* Sometimes you just have to satisfy that sweet tooth, but you can try eating fruit instead of the gooey sweet roll, or you could have cookies on hand that are made with honey, molasses, or bananas. Sugar has no nutritional benefit, and hastens tooth decay. One woman told me that she can satisfy her craving for candy by taking a teaspoon of frozen juice concentrate, for which purpose she keeps a can in the freezer already opened. For some, popcorn works.

Remember, only one change per week. At the end of the week, make one more additional change. Your second record should now reflect two changes. Continue in this way, one week at a time, until you have done all the appropriate changes. Some changes are much harder than others, and if you feel you need two or three weeks to get used to one change before trying another, that is up to you. Please don't give up after one change, or two changes. What you're after is total health improvement.

Advanced Good Eating

There are two more changes to be made after you have completed the previous seven. You can do them both at once, or you may want to do one at a time.

1. *Add whole grains to your diet.* That might include oats, cornmeal, wheat, bulgar, rice, and others you discover as you begin to read and learn about healthy eating. Most of them you will want to cook, although my family enjoys a granola made with uncooked oats, wheat bran, Grape Nuts cereal, and raisins or dates.

2. *Eliminate fat from your diet.* That is, eliminate the fat you know about. There are fats in many foods that you are not aware of, but nutritional charts will help you identify most of them. You don't need to worry about not getting enough fat. You will get fat in your food even when you try very hard not to. Read labels. Consult the chart at the end of this chapter for foods low in fat content. Then enjoy the tasty new dishes you are going to be serving.

Continue to monitor what you eat for the next month. By that time your new eating behaviors will be firmly established. During times of high stress or great temptation, return to your records. Writing things down will help you through the tough times. I'm always concerned about holidays. Our traditions of feasting are ingrained, but they don't have to be gluttonous orgies. Young children have the right idea. They are so excited about major holiday celebrations that they hardly eat a bite from the festive board. Moderation is the byword.

It may be that you are not able to follow these guidelines because of problems with your teeth and gums, or of difficulties with swallowing and digestion. If there is a problem that can be fixed, I hope you will attend to it as soon as possible. The quality of your life will be vastly improved by being able to eat normally. If your problem can't be fixed, then do the best you can to make your food more nutritious. There are vitamin and mineral supplements in liquid or powder form which you could mix into puddings and other soft foods you must eat. Fruit and vegetable juices can be included in your daily fare, perhaps as snacks. Your doctor can also advise you about a liquid supplement. Please don't give up on yourself — good nutrition makes a difference.

Exercise

Diet and exercise are like movies and popcorn: one is not complete without the other.

You can't help but improve your health if you follow the right exercise program for you and use good judgment. There are 70- and 80-year-old people who run. I have a 70-year-old friend who runs five miles every morning, and competes in 10K events. At age 60, she ran a marathon. Just the other day I read about a 100-year-old runner. And then there is Karl Oscar.

At age 60, Karl is planning a 250-mile bicycle trip over mountain passes. He has made this trip five times before. He packs a sleeping bag and food and water for three days. When night comes, he sleeps a short distance from the road, often with no shelter. Karl Oscar has a weak leg, a reminder of a bout with polio when young. Between trips, he bicycles seven miles one day and walks four the next. For Karl Oscar, keeping fit is a very high priority.

Running or biking may not be the best exercise for you, and Karl's example is extreme, but it does show that age is not a deterrent to keeping fit. The kind of exercise you do is determined by the condition of your body, not by how old you are.

Two Things Your Body Needs

There are two basic kinds of exercise: aerobic (conditioning) and toning (stretching). Both are necessary for good health. Aerobic exercise involves 20 minutes or more of sustained activity such as walking, swimming, bicycling, and dancing. It's called aerobic exercise because of the increased demand for oxygen, which is met by increased heart rate, stroke volume, respiratory rate, and relaxation of small blood vessels. This kind of exercise will strengthen your cardiovascular system and give you more energy. In order to get this conditioning effect, you need to do it three or four times a week.

Toning exercises are meant to improve muscle flexibility and joint mobility. For some people, this may be the only kind of exercise possible. For those who can do aerobic exercise, the toning exercises should be included as warm-ups before exercising, and at the end of exercise to cool down. No special equipment is needed — just loose clothes.

I know of several men and women who only do exercises in the water. Some swim laps, some do aqua aerobics, some just do range-of-motion exercises. Most pool therapy is based on knowledge of the physical properties of water, such as buoyancy and viscosity, as well as its hydrostatic and hydrodynamic properties. The temperature of the water is important, too. An individual standing neck deep in water will have an apparent weight loss of 90 percent, meaning that the feet and legs of a 130-pound person will have to support only 13 pounds. That can be a significant benefit for a person with arthritis. Studies on astronauts have shown that in the absence of gravity, the body loses lymphocytes, which have a role in the inflammatory process involved in some forms of arthritis.

The drawback to doing only water exercises is that most people need to bear weight in order to maintain or increase bone density. Unless you are medically prohibited from weight bearing, it would be best to combine water exercises with some other activity, such as walking. Pool programs are offered by community parks, universities, and some hospitals.

The right kind of exercise for you, when done in the right amount, has benefits unobtainable from any drug. In addition to the toning and conditioning effects on your heart, lungs, and muscles, exercise can clear your mind and lift depression. A 20-minute walk strengthens your bones and relieves tension. There are many opportunities for additional exercise such as climbing stairs — if you're able — instead of taking the elevator, parking your car at the far end of the parking lot, and walking around the golf course instead of using a cart. Kneading bread is a conditioning exercise. Some studies done on orchestral musicians show that pianists, string players, and conductors gain a conditioning effect from the sustained, rhythmic use of their arms. Patrick Fanning, author of *Lifetime Weight Control*, suggests more ways to increase activity:

- Walk, instead of driving, when you are going to places close by.
- Instead of using the TV remote control, get up and change the channel.
- Volunteer to do door-to-door collections for the Cancer Society, the American Lung Association, or any charity you care about.

Think of all the things you do in a day that require repetitive use of your arms and legs. It's important to be as physically active as you can be.

Grace and Tim

Grace's husband, Tim, played football in college and took up tennis as a young adult. He drifted into golf as he grew older. Tim was a little paunchy, but by following

Grace's low-fat diet, he had begun to see the return of his waistline. When Grace said she had to add exercise to her cholesterol-control program, Tim suggested they play golf together.

Grace:	That would be fun, but it has to be aerobic exercise, and we have to be able to do it year-round.
Tim:	Hey, I do a lot of walking when I golf.
Grace:	Don't you just walk a little distance and then stand around?
Tim:	Well, something like that, I guess — but still, it is walking.
Grace:	I know, dear, but the doctor said we have to do continuous exercise that gets the heart rate up to a certain level, and keeps it there for 15 minutes.
Tim:	OK, OK, what do you want to do...jog?
Grace:	Oh no, that's too hard on the knees. We could walk, or we could bicycle.
Tim:	I thought you said year-round exercise. We can't walk when there's two feet of snow on the ground.
Grace:	We can walk in the mall. There was a pamphlet in the doctor's waiting room telling about mall walking. That mall out on south 34th is exactly one mile around if you walk into every court. We could start with once around until we get used to it, and then we could go around twice. That would be two miles.
Tim:	I can add. When do we start?

Year-Round Conditioning

Remember that you are a complex person, made up of many systems. All of your inner systems depend upon each other. They are also affected by what's going on in the world around you. You already know that you can get sick from worry, fear, anxiety, and anger. Instead of worry, fear, anxiety, and anger, you can react with courage, strength, and optimism. Before doing any kind of exercise, check with your primary care doctor. Some exercises might not be good for a person who has lung and heart disease, or a connective tissue disease that is active. Although these exercises suggested here are very mild, it is best to be sure.

Mall walking is one good solution to the problem of year-round walking. No sun, no rain, no snow — just a bright and pleasant place to walk. Of course, it won't do to stop and shop since that would defeat the conditioning effect of *sustained* exercise. Resist the temptation to stop off for Aunt Agatha's birthday present. You can go back and do that *after* the walk. Malls are usually open at 7:00 a.m. for walkers when the stores are still closed, which makes it easier to resist temptation.

You can even take a walk inside the house when the weather is bad. Walk around every room in the house, and continue walking for 20 minutes. It's a little boring, but it's still exercise. To relieve the boredom, you could do a visualization, such as imagining that you are strolling through a beautiful forest or walking a country road. You could even use this walk to take note of all the things about your house that you like, and try to find just one thing you might want to take on as an improvement project. You can also walk with a portable phone and talk to your sister.

Exercise bicycles or treadmills are good, if you can afford either one. You can watch TV or listen to music. One woman told me she knits while bicycling. You might even use that time to listen to foreign language tapes. Be creative. Accept the challenge of finding ways to be on the move, rather than sitting or lying down.

Begin your walk with three minutes of stretching. Follow the example of a cat and stretch your arms, legs, and back as he does when he wakes from a nap. Start your walk at a leisurely pace, gradually increasing speed to a comfortably brisk level. After 10 minutes, stop briefly to check your heart rate. You can find your pulse at the inside of the wrist, just below the thumb; or you can feel the artery in your neck, just below the corner of your jaw. Either way will do. Count your pulse for only 10 seconds, and then multiply by 6. If you try to count for an entire minute, your heart will be slowing down, and you will interrupt the conditioning process. During the first two weeks, you should check your heart rate about three times during a 20-minute walk. At the end of the walk, start slowing down.

For optimum conditioning, you need to know your target heart rate. A target heart rate is usually indicated by two numbers, the lower one suggesting a minimum number of times per minute your heart should beat during exercise, and the higher number suggesting a maximum. To find your range, use the following formula:

Your Target Heart Rate
1. Subtract your age from 220.
2. Multiply that figure by .65 to find the lower limit.
3. Multiply the first figure by .85 to find the higher limit.

During aerobic exercise, your heart rate should remain between your two target figures for 20 minutes. You'll want to work up to that rate slowly, and come down slowly after exercise. That means taking time to warm up, and tapering off instead of stopping abruptly.

If you feel out of breath, have pain in your chest or elsewhere, slow down, and forget about the target heart rate. Please don't risk strain or injury by staying in the target rate if it is not comfortable. Your body isn't like anyone else's. If you need to walk more slowly, you will still be getting benefits from the exercise. Walking is supposed to help you feel good, not hurt you.

Whatever kind of exercise you choose, aim for *three or four times a week*, with each session lasting about *20 minutes*. That is all that is required to increase fitness. Less than that can cause more harm than good — you put sudden strain on a heart that is not properly conditioned. For this reason, also, always include a slow warm-up and cool-down period before and after each session.

If you have muscle or joint pain that comes on some time after the walk and lasts for hours, you know you have done too much. In either case, it would be well to consult your doctor or physical therapist for advice about the right kind of exercise for you.

Toning

These stretching and toning exercises can be done while you are sitting, standing, or even in the shower. I do them in the shower because the warm water helps keep my muscles relaxed. These exercises also incorporate the Feldenkrais technique of awareness through movement. Moshe Feldenkrais, a physicist, developed his techniques through application of muscle image in the motor areas of the brain. One of his ideas was that by moving your eyes, which are an extension of the brain, in the pathway you want the muscles to go, you can increase the mobility of the muscles.

Read through each exercise. Before you move any muscles, close your eyes. Now let your eyes move slowly through the pathway your head (arm, leg, and so forth) is going to go. For example, if you are going to move your chin down to your chest, first close your eyes and move your eyes downward as if they were looking at the spot on your chest where your chin is going. Do this two more times. Then go ahead with the exercise.

Do these exercises slowly, stopping if you feel pain. Never push beyond discomfort — you could hurt yourself. And remember to *breathe*. Inhale deeply before you begin, then exhale during the movement. Sometimes people get so involved in trying to remember what to move where that they fail to breathe. Muscles need a constant supply of oxygen in order to do the work you're asking them to do. The only way they get it is if you breathe.

Shoulder Shrugs

1. Straighten your posture before you begin.
2. Lift your shoulders up and back as far as you can, using a circular motion. Breathe in as you move. Exhale at the end of the movement.
3. Now roll your shoulders forward and down in the same kind of circle. Breathe as you did for the backward roll.
4. Repeat 2 times, and work up to 5 repetitions over a period of four weeks.

Shoulder Circles

1. Circle your right shoulder up, forward, and down, breathing deeply. Now do the same circle up, back, and down.
2. Do these 2 circles with the left shoulder.
3. Repeat twice, and work up to 5 over a period of four weeks.

Elbow Circles

1. Place your fingertips on your shoulders.
2. Rotate your shoulders in backward circles. Make a very small circle at first. If that is comfortable, you may try a slightly larger circle. If it hurts anywhere, stop, or go back to a smaller circle. Repeat 3 times, or as many as feels comfortable. Please remember to breathe.
3. Rotate your shoulders in small forward circles, as you did in step 2.

Arm Circles

1. Extend your arms out to the sides with your hands flexed upward as if you had your palms pressed against two walls.
2. Make small circles with your arms, first forward and then back. If there is no discomfort, you can increase the size of the circles. Do this 3 times.

Head Rolls

1. Sitting straight with your hands on your knees, lower your chin to your chest. Rest there for 3 counts.
2. Roll your right ear to your shoulder for 3 counts. Most likely your ear will not touch your shoulder; you're just going in that direction.
3. Now return to center, and tilt your head backwards until you can look at the ceiling. Return to center.
4. Repeat step 2 to the left, keeping your left ear to your left shoulder for 3 counts.
5. Now do a slow right connected motion — right ear to right shoulder, chin to chest, left ear to left shoulder, chin to chest, right ear to right shoulder. It is not a good idea to roll your head all the way around because it stresses the facet joints. Are you breathing?

Arm Reaches

1. Place your chair near a wall, or stand at arm's length from the wall.
2. Place your right palm flat against the wall. Crawl up the wall as high as you can comfortably reach. Hold that position for 3 to 5 counts. Let your hand slide back down the wall.

3. Turn and do the same with your left hand and arm.

Elbow to Knee

1. Place your hands behind your head.
2. Take a deep breath.
3. As you exhale, bend forward and twist so that your right elbow goes toward your left knee. Just go as far as you can without pain or strain.
4. Return to the straight position, breathe in deeply.
5. Breathe out and bend with your left elbow going toward your right knee. Please do all of these movements slowly, breathing in deeply before you bend and breathing out as you bend. 2 or 4 repetitions is enough for the first two weeks. You will never need to do more than 5.

This same movement may be repeated with a shoulder-to-knee action. Only do this if it is comfortable. There are other twisting exercises which will not be included here. The potential for back injury is greater when twisting if it is not carefully done. If you wish more of that kind of exercise, first consult your doctor about the condition of your spine. Then look at one of the books listed at the end of the chapter, or check your library under fitness and exercise; your doctor might also have suggestions.

Bent Leg Lift

1. Sit on the edge of your chair in a good posture.
2. Hold the side of the chair with your hands. Your knees are bent.
3. Lift one leg, hold for 3 counts, and lower. Repeat with the other leg. Try 3 repetitions for a while, and then, if comfortable, work up to 5 to 7. Remember to breathe in, then exhale while lifting your leg.

Bend and Breathe I

1. Sit on the edge of your chair in a good posture.
2. Have your feet flat on the floor in front of you, in line with your hips.
3. Take a deep breath.
4. As you exhale, bend slowly forward and let your hands slide down your legs until they rest on top of your feet.
5. Remain there, breathing normally, for 5 counts. Then return to a sitting position.

Bend and Breathe II

1. Sit on the chair as before with your feet on the floor, lined up with your hips.
2. Take a deep breath.
3. As you exhale, bend slowly forward and place your hands flat on the floor between your feet.

4. Remain there, breathing normally, for 5 counts. Return to a sitting position.

Those last two exercises are marvelous if you have twitchy legs. Some people call them "restless legs." It's the unbearable twitches you feel in your legs after sitting for a long time, or when you lie down at night to go to sleep. No one seems to have a very good explanation for it, and doctors sometimes prescribe muscle relaxants, which can, unfortunately, lead to a drug misuse habit. Instead of that, try the exercises, unless there is some reason why you can not assume this position.

Range of Motion

Putting all of your joints through a range of motions every day is important in order to avoid stiffness and loss of function. You have already done that with your head and shoulders. Most of these can be done sitting or lying down. I have not included many standing exercises because it is easier to get into trouble with those. If you are agile and want to do standing or seated floor exercises, you could consult any book on yoga. You could even take a class, and that would give you an opportunity to meet new people. Feldenkrais has excellent exercises in his book, *Awareness Through Movement*, and there are video tapes available. You just need to know what your limitations are, and what is safe and beneficial for you to do.

Remember to follow through the motions in your mind, with your eyes closed, before you begin. Feldenkrais says that this will open the pathways your muscles will follow.

1. While sitting, perhaps as you watch television or travel, place your feet flat on the floor and move one at a time in an upward motion, keeping your heel on the floor, bending at the ankle.
2. If that goes well, draw small circles in the air with your feet. Your heals stay on the ground.
3. Stand at a counter, steady yourself with your hands, and rise up on your toes. (One of the reasons I keep cautioning you about limitation is that I know a woman who went up on her toes and broke three bones in her foot. She has osteoporosis, a condition that can impose quite a few limitations.)
4. Stand sideways to a counter or table. Steady yourself with a hand, and slowly, always slowly, raise your outside leg straight to the front. Go only as far as is comfortable. Hold for 3 counts, and gently lower it.
5. Do the same with the other leg.
6. Now raise your leg straight out to the side.
7. Do the same with the other leg.

For steps 8 through 10 you need equipment. A cut-off broom handle the length of the distance between your shoulders will work, and so will a cane or a two-inch dowel from the lumber yard.

8. Lie down on your back with a pillow under your knees. Grasp the broom handle or cane with both hands, palms facing away from you. Now raise it slowly up and back so that your arms extend back over your head. You don't need to straighten them completely: just enough so you feel a stretch. Bring the handle slowly back to eye-level and repeat 3 times. Do this motion *slowly,* and smoothly. Stop if you feel pain.

9. Now bring the cane down to your chest. Raise it straight up the way a weight lifter does. If it's comfortable, do it 3 times. Are you breathing?

10. Now raise the cane straight up again and make a semi-circle in the air, keeping your arms straight. Do that 3 times if it feels OK. Do this slowly and gently, and stop if anything hurts. Some people can do this exercise when they can't do the shoulder and elbow rolls. After several months, you can fasten a one-pound weight to the center of the cane. More weight than that is not necessary.

11. Make small circles in the air with your hands, bending at the wrists.

12. Bend your elbows 3 times.

Total Health

And finally, a summary of suggestions on how to become as totally, wholly healthy as you can be.

1. Make food preparation an act of love. Choose foods that will give strength and promote wellness. This week, experiment with three new recipes (following the food guidelines given at the beginning of the chapter. As you will notice on the chart that follows, many low-fat foods are also high in fiber.

2. Exercise aerobically at least three times a week. Choose an exercise that is right for your body. Take your first steps today.

3. Include toning exercises in your daily routine to maintain strength and flexibility.

4. Listen to what your body is telling you about your state of wellness. Respect pain and other symptoms, but don't become obsessed with them.

References

American Honey Institute. (1945) *Old Favorite Honey Recipes.* Madison, WI.

Birkedahl, N. (1990) *The Habit Control Workbook.* Oakland, CA: New Harbinger Publications, Inc.

Davis, M., E.R. Eshelman, and M. McKay, (1980) *The Relaxation & Stress Reduction Workbook.* Oakland, CA: New Harbinger Publications, Inc.

Evans, R.L. (1971) *Richard Evan's Quote Book.* Salt Lake City: Publishers Press.

Feldenkrais, M. (1977) *Awareness Through Movement.* New York: Harper and Row.

Fanning, P. (1990) *Lifetime Weight Control.* Oakland, CA: New Harbinger Publications, Inc.

Larson, D., ed. (1990) *Mayo Clinic Family Health Book.* New York: William Morrow and Company, Inc.

"Boning up on Osteoporosis" (1989) National Osteoporosis Foundation, in conjunction with the Osteoporosis Center, University of Connecticut Health Center.

Vithoulkas, G. (1980) *The Science of Homeopathy.* New York: Grove Press.

Pritikin, R. (1990) *The New Pritikin Program.* New York: Simon & Schuster.

Diet, Nutrition, and Cancer Prevention. United States Department of Health and Humanities.

Nutrition Chart: Fats and Fiber

Low-Fat Foods:

Apples
Acerola
Alfalfa sprouts
Apples
Artichokes
Barley, pearled
Beans (green, red, navy, black)
Brown rice
Berries
Broccoli
Brussel sprouts
Buckwheat
Bulgur
Cabbage
Carrots
Cauliflower
Cereals, oats, wheat, rice
Cherries
Chicken
Cottage cheese (low-fat)
Cowpeas
Greens (spinach, kale, beet greens, etc.)
Kiwi
Leeks
Lentils
Lettuce
Melons
Oranges
Parsnips
Pasta
Peaches
Pears
Peas
Plantain
Potatoes
Squash
Tomatoes
Turnips

High-Fiber Foods:

Bananas
Barley
Beans (dry)
Berries
Bran, wheat, oat
Bread
Brussel sprouts
Carrots
Cereals (ready-to-eat)
Chickpeas
Cowpeas
Figs
Greens
Millet
Papaya
Parsnips
Pears
Peas
Plantain
Prunes
Pumpkin
Winter squash

6

Managing Stress

Stress has long been a part of your life. At times it's kept you going, helping you produce and create and keep moving. At times it's been harmful, resulting in exhaustion, ill health, and painful anxiety. How you respond to stress has enormous consequences for both your emotional and physical well-being. You can't eliminate all stress from your life — the resulting boredom would be stressful — but you can learn better ways to respond to stress. The techniques in this chapter can help you recognize the current stresses in your life, and minimize the pain and anxiety they can cause. Whether you're aware of stress or not, you can only benefit from mastery of relaxation techniques. Sometimes they just help you feel better; sometimes they avert disaster.

Jane

Until 1980, Marvin's and Jane's lives had been full. Their four children were grown and established with families and careers of their own. Marvin retired from his position as superintendent of schools, and Jane, 10 years younger, continued to excel in the field of commercial art. They didn't think much about stress, although they'd had plenty of it. Daily stresses, major emergencies, and minor crises were an expected part of living, something they just dealt with and then went on. For the most part, they had enjoyed good health. Their combined income allowed them to live comfortably, educate their children, and enjoy a few luxuries, such as a motor home and a small sailboat. Then something happened to change their lives dramatically.

Shortly after Marvin retired, Jane began to have episodes of shortness of breath, rapid heartbeat, and a feeling of panic. It started one day in the grocery store where Jane often stopped after work to pick up a few items. As she walked along the aisles, picking up a jar of salsa, a package of tortillas, and other items, she noticed that she couldn't get a deep breath. It felt like there wasn't room in her lungs for more air. She kept taking deeper and deeper breaths, but she couldn't get enough air. She felt frightened, and noticed the rapid beating of her heart. Abandoning the idea of further shopping, she went to the check-out counter, feeling more shaky with every passing moment. As she stood in line, she was suddenly overwhelmed with the need to get outside, get air, get away from the crowded store. Leaving her cart, she ran out and stood by her car, sucking in great gulps of air. There was no use going back in for the groceries, she thought. Fearing she might be having a heart attack, she drove to the emergency room. She was ushered into a gown, weighed, given oxygen, and plastered with electrodes for an electrocardiogram. A doctor came in to examine her.

Doctor:	Frankly, Jane, I don't hear anything unusual in your chest, and your EKG strips are normal. Let's take off the oxygen and have you breathe into this paper bag. You may be just hyperventilating little bit.

Jane began to feel better after a few minutes of breathing into the bag. Her heart rate slowed, and she no longer felt the hunger for air.

Jane:	I don't understand this. How could this happen?
Doctor:	Stress can do it. What was your work day like?
Jane:	About usual, I guess, except...oh yes, there was an angry customer and I have to scratch a big project and start over. That's stressful, but it's happened before. It never bothered me, it's just part of the business.
Doctor:	Mmm hmm. Anything else going on in your life?
Jane:	My husband just retired, so that changes our life a bit. He's not unhappy. He's just restless, hasn't figured out what he wants to do now.
Doctor:	And the children?
Jane:	All doing fine. Our daughter is expecting her second baby, and I'm planning to be with her. That's in about a month.
Doctor:	Are you looking forward to that?
Jane:	Well, sure I am. I mean I'm looking forward to being with her, and I'll love the baby. But I guess I am a little anxious about the cost of the trip. We never used to think twice about a trip, but with our income reduced it's not easy. It doesn't seem like that would be something to get in a big tizzy about, though. It's just one of those things we have to adjust to.

The doctor turned to the nurse who was removing electrodes from Jane's chest. "Would you please bring a glass of water and some ice cubes on the side?"

Jane wondered if breathing in a bag and drinking ice water was all the treatment she was going to get. She was beginning to feel a little foolish and chagrined by her behavior. "I've always been a calm person," she thought, "I don't get upset by little things."

The doctor took the glass and asked Jane to hold it. Then he took an ice cube. "Jane, this glass of water represents the stress in your life. Everyone has stress, but everyone also has a limit to how much stress they can handle before it affects them adversely. You've been handling stress marvelously well for many years. Now," he said, putting an ice cube into the glass, "you've reached the limit." Water spilled over onto Jane's lap. The doctor laughed and took the glass.

"Sorry about that," he said, "but this is the way stress works. You handle stress as you go along, but eventually you may get too much. It only takes one stressful event too many for things to overflow and give you a shock, just like the shock of the cold water on your lap." The doctor went to the sink and poured out half the water, returning the glass to Jane. "Now, when I put in an ice cube — one more stress — the glass doesn't overflow. You can handle another stress when the glass is half full. The trick is to manage your life so that your glass never gets full enough to overflow."

That wasn't the end of Jane's panic attacks. The difference was that now she understood why they were happening and she didn't need to become frightened that she might have some life-threatening illness. She started a self-help program of stress management, and over time the attacks became less frequent and severe. Eventually they faded away entirely.

The additional stresses which triggered Jane's panic reaction were not big crises. They were small, predictable events similar to many she had experienced throughout her life. They were just too many. These small stresses filled Jane's glass of stress too full, and something had to give. She had exceeded her level of tolerance.

Not everyone reacts to stress with panic attacks. Sometimes people develop new allergies, have accidents, or develop itchy rashes. In fact, every ailment known to man, including those which are genetic, can be triggered by stress, can be made worse by stress, and can be improved by reducing stress. And that's what this chapter aims to do: help you learn to manage stress.

Counting Ice Cubes

Before you can effectively control stress, you need to recognize the specific stresses in your life. You have to see which ice cubes are too much for a full glass. It's all a matter of cause and effect.

Hans Selye, the grandfather of stress research, defined what he called the "General Adaptation Syndrome" (GAS) in this way: *General* refers to the fact that your whole body reacts to stress; Adaptation means that you are trying to adjust all body systems to this new and difficult state; *Syndrome* means that all the manifestations of the stress reaction are coordinated and interdependent. Another way to say it would be, you are trying your best to get used to a bad situation and it causes physical and emotional symptoms. How often when you've received shocking news have you said, "That makes me sick?" You may also have heard the expression, "What a pain in the neck." Everyone's vocabulary is littered with verbal expressions related to a stress response. Isn't it bizarre to think you should be too strong to be affected by stress?

One homeopathic physician, George Vithoulkas, says that symptoms of any kind indicate that the body's defense mechanism is doing its best to heal. The symptoms are not problems in themselves; they are manifestations of adjustment to trauma. Trauma can be infection, surgery, an accident, or emotional shock. It can even be from drugs, in which case symptoms are euphemistically called "side effects."

It's important to realize that your body wants to heal, and that includes mental, spiritual, and emotional healing. There are things you can do to aid the healing. Managing stress is critical, because when you become ill mentally, spiritually, or emotionally, you are in more danger than you would be from any infection or injury.

Frank

You saw how Jane reacted to ongoing and ever-increasing problems in her life. Frank's story is a little different. Frank and his sons had made a tradition of an annual hunting trip. When the sons married and had children, the grandchildren were included in these trips as soon as they were old enough to pass the hunter safety course. Frank felt good about teaching his progeny to develop good attitudes about hunting, to use their skills to obtain food, rather than to enjoy conquest. Two years ago Frank, with his four sons and three grandchildren, headed for the high country prepared for several days of camping. One son had lost his job and so they were hoping to supply his family with enough meat for the winter. The first day out, Frank took his granddaughter with him to a prearranged hunting site. The others went in different directions. It was the granddaughter who first sighted antlers just barely showing above the brush.

"Grandpa," she whispered, "I think it's a buck."

"Just wait, honey," Frank whispered back. "Let him move into the clearing. We want to make sure before we shoot." Frank shifted his weight from his stiff knee and a twig cracked. Suddenly the buck turned, charging toward them. Taken by surprise, Frank lost his balance and tumbled over. His granddaughter became confused and started to run. Frank struggled to get to his feet and dropped his rifle. The buck stopped, turned toward Frank, and then veered off, crashing through the brush in a different direction. The danger was over. Or was it?

Frank was sweating. He rubbed his hand across his face, aware of the heavy pounding of his heart. Then he fell to the ground. His granddaughter knelt beside him.

"What is it, Grandpa? What's wrong?"

Frank could not answer. His granddaughter fired three shots into the air, and soon help was at hand. Frank had suffered a stroke.

In the face of danger, Frank's adrenal glands had poured out massive amounts of adrenaline, making his heart beat faster, giving him energy to respond. Frank's narrowed arteries couldn't handle the challenge of the greater volume of blood being pumped through his system. An artery in his brain ruptured, causing Frank to collapse.

This "fight-or-flight" response is good if you are in sudden life-threatening danger, provided your body is in good enough shape to take it. The trouble is, you can have this same response to events that are not life-threatening, such as having prolonged, excessive medical expenses. When this is repeated over and over, the cumulative effects on your body can be disastrous.

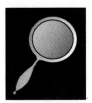 There are things you can do to be prepared for stress. First you need to identify the stresses you are facing in your life right now. For the next week, keep a record of daily events in the Ice Cube Record on the next page, marking the appropriate column to indicate the ways in which you are affected by these events. Calling these events "Ice Cubes" helps you see them objectively. Make seven copies of this record so you will have one for each day of the week. Keep one handy so that it will be easy to remember to mark. A blank chart won't do you any good.

For example, Terry awoke one morning to find that a small puddle had collected under a part of the roof that had just been fixed. He felt a surging fustration and anger, and didn't know what to do. While he considered his options, he used his Ice Cube Record to write down how he was feeling and what he was thinking. His thoughts and feelings at the time were important parts of his problem, after all.

Terry's Ice Cube Record

Date: <u>Friday, May 1</u>

Ice Cube	I felt	I said to myself	Later I had symptoms of
The roof leaked.	Angry and helpless.	Might as well give up.	Heartburn

During the day, when you feel yourself reacting to an event, jot it down on your record. Pay close attention to your body, and write in any unusual symptoms, even if they don't seem related. You may find patterns that surprise you. A later exercise will help you organize your approach to the problem situation itself. For now, you want to focus in on your body's response.

How many ice cubes did you have the first day? Write the number at the bottom of the page. Do the same with every page. Now count up how many times you had physical symptoms following an ice cube, and record those numbers. Are you surprised at the number of times you have physical symptoms after stressful events? Perhaps you are lucky and rarely have stress-induced symptoms. If that is the case, you have probably

Ice Cube Record

(make seven copies)

Date:_____

Ice Cube	I felt	I said to myself	Later I had symptoms of

Total ice cubes: _____

Typical physical reactions: _____

Frequency of physical reaction: _____

already learned how to handle stress effectively. But it can't hurt to become consciously aware of this process.

Now take a look at the "I felt" column. Is there one emotion that appears again and again? Do you respond most frequently with anger? Fear? Sadness? This is important because if you know that your most usual response is fear, for example, you can learn to spot that feeling and relate it to a recent stressful event. Then you can work on changing that fear into something less harmful and more productive.

Spotting Trouble

In World War I and II, as you will recall, there were people designated as "airplane spotters." Some were military personnel, but many were volunteers. Their job was to spend a certain number of hours watching the skies for foreign aircraft. They were especially concerned about reconnaissance planes. This was a laborious tracking system, but it worked fairly well. As radar systems became more sophisticated, the need for spotters lessened. In recent military encounters, lightning-fast computerized tracking systems allowed very specific identification of the exact nature of something traveling through the air. Not only that, the systems made it possible to intercept missiles with other missiles. Although not perfect, the new technology proved fast and accurate. It seemed almost automatic.

When you start spotting negative feelings, you will be like the airplane spotters of old. It will be a tedious, laborious process. But it won't take long for you to develop your radar system for automatic identification of feelings and the thoughts that preceded them.

You are limited, as we all are, in how much control you have over the number of ice cubes that get put in your glass. Things happen. A leaky roof might have been prevented but, on the other hand, Terry may not have been in a position to get the roof checked periodically. Since there are some things you can't control, your only recourse is to control yourself — that is, to control your reactions to events. The goal is to maintain a calm, tranquil attitude. You want to feel capable and in control. You want to keep your stress glass only half full so that one more ice cube won't hurt.

In order to do that, you have to spot the feeling you get when bad things happen. Then you have to identify the words you said to yourself during the moment *before* the feeling. Think back to Chapter 3, where you learned about feelings and self-talk with regard to self-esteem. Those principles apply now to threatening events.

Frank's first thought when the buck came charging was, "He'll kill Emily!" Then, when he was having trouble getting up, he thought, "Oh no, I can't, I'm stuck," followed by, "Stupid old fool."

Every statement enhanced his total body response to the threat. All kinds of biochemical changes were taking place in a matter of seconds. Had he been aware of his self-defeating response, he might have been able to encounter it with a self-affirming response. Remember your Spot and Stop Record, where you rewrote negative statements into healthy, accurate ones? You want to do the same thing in stressful situations, harnessing your mind's ability to influence your body. Ideally, you want to create a calm, rational state instead of an anxious one. Do you see any statements on your Ice Cube Record that you might rewrite into healthier, more accurate statements? Now is a good time to look back.

Controlling your body's responses until you have achieved a degree of calm frees you to address the crisis itself. There was a reason, after all, you began to feel stress. It may be that the crisis demands an immediate response; in this case, you depend on your own reflexes and common sense. A habit of viewing sudden proceedings with calm, and of trusting your own ability to act, will prepare you to handle such situations. That's what Frank needed, but failed to find in his moment of panic. In most crisis situations, fortunately, you will have some time to assess your alternatives. Just as in any problem-solving model, the best approach is to view the situation objectively, brainstorm possible solutions, and evaluate them rationally. The Crisis Worksheet on the following page can help you do this.

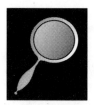 Make several copies of the blank crisis worksheet before you begin, so you can use it for future crises. Then pick one problem currently causing you stress, and write it on the top of the worksheet. If you like, pick one problem from your Ice Cube Record. Begin with the first column, Options List, and write down every possible solution you can think of, no matter how crazy it seems. When you have written at least five, fill in the second column, asking yourself "Who can help." You may want to ask someone for advice or actual assistance, or you may prefer to resolve the crisis alone. Next, fill in the Cost column, considering emotional and physical costs as well as financial. Only when you have written and considered all the options you can think of, turn to the last column. Based on the objective information you see, and your subjective feeling, decide whether or not the resolution is possible.

For example, Donna's car insurance rate went up recently, without any increase in her income. She felt very anxious about the situation, and finally decided to stop forcing it out of her mind and to face it rationally.

Donna found the very act of working out a solution to be calming. Uncertainty and indecisiveness were driving her crazy. Take a look at what Donna wrote on her Crisis Worksheet on the page following the blank worksheet.

You can see that Donna has a sense of humor, which is a wonderful way to take the tragedy out of any situation. I doubt if she seriously considered becoming a bag lady, although I did read a delightful novel about a woman who did just that. Spend some time working on solutions for some of the problems you've encountered recently. Before Donna started the worksheet, she would have considered selling the car an impossible choice, but as she contemplated all possible solutions, that choice didn't seem so bad.

The next challenge in stress management is to develop control over your body's response to stress. There are many methods for training your mind and body to stay relaxed, happy, and calm. When your muscles are relaxed, your mind will be calm. When your mind is calm, your muscles relax. The relaxation techniques described below can help replace a negative thought-and-feeling pattern with a pattern that keeps positive energy flowing. When you can interrupt your body's physical response to stress, both body and mind will benefit.

Crisis Worksheet

Problem:

Options List:	Who Can Help:	Cost:	Yes/No
1.			
2.			
3.			
4.			
5.			
6.			
7.			
8.			

Final Solution:

Donna's Crisis Worksheet

Problem: I don't have enough money to pay the car insurance.

Options List:	Who Can Help:	Cost:	Yes/No
1. Not pay.	No one.	Illegal.	No, won't do.
2. Pay part.	Insurance agent.	Small fine.	Yes, could work.
3. Borrow.	Son.	Shame.	Last resort.
4. Become bag lady.	Only me.	Too high.	No, ridiculous.
5. Sell car.	Mr. Evans.	Be on foot.	Next to last resort.

Final Solution: Talk to insurance agent about making two or three payments instead of one. It will probably only cost three or four dollars more. Since it's illegal to drive without insurance, I hope this works. If not, I'll talk to Mr. Evans about selling the car. It's not the end of the world to be without a car. I might even look into possibilities for increasing my monthly income.

Melting Ice Cubes

If you keep your body at its peak, you will have reserves of energy to handle stress. The diet and exercise guidelines mentioned in the previous chapter are important components of a good health and anti-stress program. Your reserves won't be there if you're tired out, malnourished, and flabby. Stress also requires some specialized exercises. Some of the exercises that follow ensure long-term improvements in your body's responses to stress. Others provide "on-the-spot" relief when panic threatens to strike.

Yoga and Deep Breathing

Annie Besant, in her little book, *An Introduction to Yoga*, describes the practice of yoga in this way. The gardener uses intelligence to select plants that have qualities he desires, and then he places pollen from the chosen plant upon the carpels of another. He does not leave pollination to the bees. The gardener repeats this process until he has produced a flower so different from its original stock that you can't tell where it came from.

Yoga is a system of change. It helps you unfold levels of consciousness. You become what you want to be. The ultimate aim of practicing yoga is mind control. It can help you direct your thoughts so that solutions to your problems come from your own inner wisdom. Yoga is one path to achieving mind/body balance.

Yoga begins with proper breathing. Your posture may not be the best it could be. Over the years you have probably begun to bend forward. When you do that, you restrict your ability to breathe deeply. When you don't breathe deeply, you don't sleep well, you are not as mentally alert, and you feel stiffer when lying in bed at night. Here are two breathing exercises. The first will work for anyone; the second won't do if you have painful knee, wrist, or shoulder joints.

Deep Breathing I

1. Lie down on your bed, or on the floor if you can. Lie on your back, bend your knees, and place your feet comfortably apart. Let your knees lean against each other. If your knees feel tender, place a pillow between them. Let both hands rest on your abdomen.
2. Purse your lips into an "O" and slowly push all the air from your lungs. Feel your chest and abdomen go down.
3. Inhale through your nose as if you were filling a paper bag, air going into the bottom of the bag first. You will feel your hands rise as your abdomen rises. Keep breathing in until your chest is expanded with air. As you get to the top, be sure your abdomen stays relaxed, full, and rounded.
4. Hold your breath for a short moment.
5. Purse your lips and begin to breathe out air from the top part of your lungs, slowly, slowly. As your chest and ribs cave in, tighten your abdomen inward to push out all the remaining air.
6. Continue to breathe in this way, concentrating on the breathing and nothing else. Feel your hands move up and down in regular measures, as your lungs fill and empty completely. Take 10 deep breaths this way, feeling worry and stress blow out, and good, cleansing oxygen rush in.

Deep Breathing II

1. Get into an all-fours position. It is best to do this exercise on a firm surface, but if your bed doesn't sag, you could do it there.
2. Breathe in, letting your abdomen drop, arching your back slightly, and looking upward as far as your neck will comfortably allow. Don't strain. Pain is not useful.
3. After you have inhaled completely, lower your head and look down as you forcibly blow all the air out through your nose.
4. Before breathing in again, press downward with your arms and shoulders and arch your back into a curved bridge. Pull your abdomen in and hold for a few seconds.
5. Relax now and let everything sag. Return to the first position and repeat the breathing cycle. Do this twice daily for several weeks, and then increase to three sessions. More than five is unnecessary and could even be to your disadvantage. Don't do this exercise at all if it causes pain at the time or later.

There are several other ways to do breathing exercises. These may be found in books listed at the end of the chapter. *Easy Does It Yoga for Older People* by Alice Christensen and David Rankin is one I like, as is *The Relaxation and Stress Reduction Workbook* by Martha Davis, Elizabeth Eshelman, and Matthew McKay. The following exercise is one you can do on the spot, whenever you feel tense, angry, or afraid. These exercises are useful when you can't sleep and when you are having anxious thoughts. I have found breathing exercises to be better than drugs when I wake up in the night with stiff, painful joints and muscles. This is adapted from *The Relaxation and Stress Reduction Workbook*. You can do it anywhere.

The Relaxing Sigh

The sound I hear as I walk down the hall of a nursing home is sighing, often accompanied by a small sound, something like "Ah." The next thing is a yawn. I yawn a lot myself when I'm sitting at the computer. Yawns and sighs tell you that you are not getting enough oxygen. A sigh releases tension and the yawn helps you breathe more deeply. You know how to breathe deeply now, but you may find it helpful to relieve anxiety and tension by sighing purposefully.

1. Sit or stand straight. If you are lying down, assume a position that will allow your rib cage to expand easily, as was described in the previous exercise.
2. Sigh deeply, even noisily if that feels best. Enjoy the feeling of relief as the air rushes out of your lungs.
3. Don't think about inhaling...just let the air come in as it will.
4. Repeat this process several times and as often as you need to.

Yoga and Meditation: Progressive Relaxation

Of course you know you should be able to "just relax." Everyone knows that — at least everyone talks about it — but not everyone knows how to do it. Yoga combines relaxation with meditation. Abundant research shows that this combination reduces blood pressure, eliminates pain, and has a positive effect on your biochemistry. It also gives you conscious control over the state of your muscles and your mind.

The following exercise works best if you do it at the same time every day. It will not work as well if you have been smoking, drinking caffeinated or alcoholic drinks, or if you are sedated with tranquilizers, pain pills, or sleeping aids. It's best to do it when your tummy is not too full. Pets, children, telephones, and doorbells can distract and disrupt. Plan your relaxation/meditation time so that these distractions are not present. Put the phone under a pillow and let the answering machine take messages, or else just turn the phone off. (Don't forget to turn it on again later!) Put a "Sleeping" sign on your doorbell, and solicit cooperation from your family. It's a good idea to tape the following instruction since it's distracting to have to refer to a printed page. When you are taping, read slowly, pausing for breaths at commas, and perhaps a longer pause for periods.

Lie down on your back, or rest in a reclining chair. In order to protect your back, place a pillow or two under your knees. In fact, use pillows wherever you need them in order to be comfortable. Tell yourself that for the next 10 minutes you are going to be completely relaxed and silent. Close your eyes and breathe deeply.

Focus your attention on the top of your head, where tiny muscles lace across your scalp. These muscles are tense. Tell them to let go...relax. Now do the same for muscles around your ears and in your face. Let your eyelids relax...and then let the looseness spread deeply into your eyes. Let them be still, loose, free. Now unclench the muscles around your mouth and jaw...let them go. Relax your tongue and the muscles that hold your mouth shut...let them go.

Focus on your shoulders: feel the tension that has accumulated there. Tell your shoulders to let go...to be limp, warm, and soft. Let them lie back limply, supported by the bed or chair. Now let your upper arms go...and relax your forearms and feel your hands grow heavy and limp. Your arms have become like the arms of a sleeping baby, limp, soft, warm. Your hands curl naturally, limply, as they do in sleep.

Let your awareness move now to your chest. Feel how your lungs breathe for you. You need not make any effort to breathe. Asleep or awake your lungs just keep breathing for you...in...out...in...out. Your heart beats all by itself. You don't do a thing to make it beat. Sometimes it beats fast, sometimes slow. Once in a while it skips a beat or gives an extra beat. This is normal. Everyone's heart does these things. Take time to appreciate your heart. Let the muscles in your chest grow limp so that your heart and lungs have greater freedom.

Tell your stomach and abdomen to let go now, to be limp...no need to hold things in...let everything grow flabby and soft...totally let go. Just let everything inside you happen the way it wants to. Let go and rest.

Now your legs.... Let them become limp, soft, and warm, just like a baby's legs. Tell your feet to let go...to rest, relax. Feel the warmth in your legs going to the bones...warming, strengthening the bones. Feel the warmth move up the bones in your legs to your pelvic bones and your spine. Tell the muscles to be limp so that the loose spine can align itself. See your spine from the base of your skull hanging downward like a chain. Move upward to the inside of your head. By looking at your eyes and face from the inside, you can tell if everything is relaxed and limp. Take time to let your eyes, face, neck, and shoulders become even more limp, warm, and soft. Now you can begin your meditation.

Hum the sound "om." It is an easy sound to make and does not require tensing of your mouth. Repeat "om" over and over without any effort to control loudness or softness. Just however it comes out is fine. Thoughts will enter your mind. Let them pass on through. Give them no attention. Simply be silent in your mind, bringing your attention back to "om." Everyone's thoughts wander. Just let the thoughts go and come back to "om."

You will improve every day in your ability to stay focused only on "om." You can continue with "om" for 5 to 10 minutes or you can begin to focus on prayer or another thought that has meaning for you. Savor this peace and relaxed concentration. When you are ready to come out of meditation, just gradually let your mind leave the silence as you breathe a little faster and move your arms around. Stretch the way a cat does when he wakes up. Then open your eyes, look around, and rest a few minutes before getting up. When you do get up, you will feel alert and refreshed. Your energy level will be recharged and you can go about your tasks more efficiently. Practice meditation every day. A good time would be early morning before arising, or mid-afternoon when you feel you have run out of gas for the day.

On-the-Spot Muscle Relaxation

The system with the best track record for helping people to use their minds for creating a relaxation response is called Autogenic Training (AT). You can train your body to respond to stress in a way that will prevent illness. The originator of this method was Johannes H. Schulz, a psychiatrist. *Genos* is a Greek word that means *developed. Auto means from within the self; thus autogenic means that you train yourself to evoke* psychological and physiological changes.

Schulz developed six standard exercises, and these same six exercises which Schulz used for 40 or more years with success are still used today by health professionals. The purpose of autogenic training is to promote adequate and healthy reactions of the body and the mind through relaxation, self-regulation of autonomic functions, self-determination, and insight into the inner self for self-critique and self-control.

The word *training* lets you know that this is a step-by-step process and that it is going to take time. Some of the effects noticed after two weeks might include greater relaxation, reduced anxiety, better sleep, improved memory, and greater motivation. These are all effects that increase your ability to handle stress.

This is the way it works. The conditioning effects of regular practice bring about a compulsion to complete an act. When you learned to read, you conditioned yourself to automatically recognize certain groups of letters as words. After practicing autogenic training, you will be conditioned to respond to stress with calmness, with rational thought, and without the adverse biochemical changes that have formerly made you ill.

Because of its powerful effects, you should have a physical exam and discuss the effects of AT with your doctor. If you have high or low blood pressure, be aware that it will be affected, so monitoring of your blood pressure is necessary. If you have a serious disease such as diabetes, hypoglycemia, or a heart condition, you should be supervised by your doctor. If you experience anxiety or any other unpleasant effects that don't go away, it would be better for you to work with an experienced AT trainer.

How To Do the Exercises

For AT you need the same quiet environment that you had for meditation. Wear comfortable clothing and choose a comfortable chair or bed. If you lie on your back, you will probably want pillows under your knees to prevent back stiffness when you get up. Use pillows for your neck and arms if you need them to be comfortable. Your arms should lie beside you, elbows comfortably flexed, and hands palms-down.

If you choose an armchair or a lounge chair, adjust yourself so that you feel no tension anywhere in your body. Use pillows or rolled up towels to increase comfort. Rest your arms on the chair arms, and place your feet flat on the floor or recline the chair.

As you go through the exercises, you will experience various physical and emotional changes. These are called "autogenic discharges" and will disappear as you get farther into the program. Some of these changes will be pleasant, such as feeling warm or exceptionally happy. Other changes may not be pleasant, such as pain, anxiety, headache, and others. Just say to yourself, "This is temporary," and go on with the exercise.

When you are ready to stop a session, say, "When I open my eyes, I will feel refreshed and alert." Then open your eyes, breathe deeply, yawn, and stretch. Take time to become fully awake and oriented before you get up and go about your daily tasks.

You're going to practice one part at a time, adding to it each week. Do you remember your first piano lesson? You were given *one* simple thing to practice for a week, weren't you? The second week you practiced the first thing as well as one more thing, and so on. And that's the way Van Cliburn got to Carnegie Hall.

Let your mind be open and receptive to whatever will happen. Don't set up expectations or goals. Just erase your thoughts and let go. When distracting thoughts creep in, just let them float on through. This is called "passive concentration." Are you ready?

Basic Autogenic Training

Practice each week's formula once or twice a day for the full week before moving on to the next level.

1. Heaviness Theme

Week 1: Repeat this formula slowly 6 times:

My right arm is heavy.

My left arm is heavy.

Both arms are very heavy.

Now say "Tranquil" 1 time.

Wait a few seconds and breathe deeply before repeating the formula.

Week 2: Repeat slowly 6 times:

My right arm is heavy.

My left arm is heavy.

Both arms are very heavy.

My right leg is heavy.

My left leg is heavy.
Both arms and legs are very heavy.
Say "Tranquil" once.
Wait and breathe.

Week 3: Repeat slowly 6 times:
My right arm is heavy.
Both of my arms are heavy.
Both of my legs are heavy.
My arms and legs are very heavy.
Say "Tranquil" once.
Wait and breathe.

2. *Warmth Theme*
Week 4: Repeat 6 times, slowly:
My right arm is heavy.
My arms and legs are heavy.
My right arm is warm.
My left arm is warm.
Both of my arms are warm.
Say "Tranquil" once.
Wait and breathe.

You can use visual imagery if you have difficulty feeling the warmth and heaviness. Picture yourself in a tub of hot water, or imagine a heating pad placed upon your arms or legs. You can also visualize yourself lying in the sun with your head in the shade of a tree.

Week 5: Repeat 6 times, slowly:
My right arm is heavy.
My arms and legs are heavy.
My right arm is warm.
My left arm is warm.
My right leg is warm.
My left leg is warm.
Both of my legs are warm.
My arms and legs are warm.
Say "Tranquil" once.
Wait and breathe.

Week 6: Repeat 6 times, slowly:
My right arm is heavy.
My arms and legs are very heavy.
My right arm is warm.
Both of my arms are warm.
My right leg is warm.

Both of my legs are warm.
My arms and legs are warm.
My arms and legs are heavy and warm.
Say "Tranquil" once.
Wait and breathe.

Week 7: Repeat 6 times, slowly:
My right arm is heavy.
My arms and legs are very heavy.
My right arm is warm.
My arms and legs are warm.
My arms and legs are heavy and warm.
Say "Tranquil" once.
Wait and breathe.

3. *Heartbeat Theme*
Week 8: Repeat 6 times, slowly:
My right arm is heavy and warm.
My arms and legs are heavy and warm.
My heartbeat is calm and regular.
Say "Tranquil" once.
Wait and breathe.

4. *Breathing Theme*
Week 9: Repeat 6 times, slowly:
My right arm is heavy and warm.
My arms and legs are heavy and warm.
My heartbeat is calm and regular.
It breathes me.
Say "Tranquil" once.
Wait and breathe.

5. *Solar Plexus Theme*
Week 10: Only do this exercise if you do *not* have ulcers, diabetes, or any condition involving bleeding from abdominal organs. Repeat 6 times, slowly:
My right arm is heavy and warm.
My arms and legs are heavy and warm.
My heartbeat is calm and regular.
It breathes me.
My solar plexus is warm.
Say "Tranquil" once.
Wait and breathe.

6. *Forehead Theme*
Week 11: Repeat 6 times, slowly:
My right arm is heavy and warm.

> My arms and legs are heavy and warm.
> My heartbeat is calm and regular.
> It breathes me.
> My solar plexus is warm.
> My forehead is cool.
> Say "Tranquil" once.
> Wait and breathe.

This last segment is the one you can use on a daily basis, as regularly as brushing your teeth. It takes about 7 to 10 minutes, but you will experience the benefits all day long. You can also use it when you feel yourself getting upset or when a crisis occurs. For quick help in an emergency, just say "Tranquility," and all the good effects of AT will be there.

Visualization

The more tricks you have in your bag the better. Yoga, meditation, and exercise are ongoing affairs. Paying attention to your nutritional requirements is a daily and never-ending concern. But why not learn a few special techniques that you can pull out for unexpected stresses? During the hard times it's easy to get burned out, harried, frantic, and find yourself out of control.

Recently I went to hear the Concordia College Singers, who were touring our area. They sang a spiritual that had a powerful message. I plan to write the words on a card and place it where I can read it often. This is what they sang:

> Slow me down, Lord, I'm going too fast;
>   Can't see my brother when he's goin' past.
> Miss a lot of good things, day by day;
>   Won't know a blessing when it comes my way.
> Everybody's rushing all around! Slow me down, Lord, slow me down.

The best thing you can do when emergencies seem to come in a continuous stream, piling up in the most intimidating way, is to slow down. Visualization is one way to do that. You daydream sometimes, don't you? You find yourself thinking about something that happened a long time ago, remembering details and the feelings. Or perhaps you daydream about something you would like to do. You imagine yourself having conversations with interesting people, or growing a lovely rose garden. It can be as real as if it were really happening. That's visualization. You didn't have to learn to do that, it's a natural thing. Since you already have this skill, you just need to learn how to make it work for you.

Patrick Fanning, in his book, *Visualization for Change,* defines visualization in this way: "The conscious, volitional creation of mental sense impressions for the purpose of changing yourself." He means that visualization is something you do when you're awake, and that you do it because you have chosen to do it. He also explains that visualization is not all visual. You can hear music and voices, have an awareness of odors, feel cold or hot, and make use of all the senses. A memory is something you *re-create*. A visualization is something you *create* from scratch.

Active Versus Passive Visualization

Visualization can be passive or active. Passive, or receptive, visualization is simply a matter of clearing your mind, making it blank, and relaxing. You can then ask yourself a question about something that is of concern at the moment, and wait for an answer from your deeper mind to come to the surface. For example, you might ask yourself why you feel anxious when you read the obituaries. Besides the obvious sadness when you read about good friends who have died, you may receive an unexpected answer, such as, "Grandmother told me it was bad luck to read about people dying." You probably "forgot" that admonition a long time ago, but it still affects you.

Active visualization is like writing a script for a play. You plan what you want to feel, do, see, or experience, and then you see yourself going through it. Skiers do this. When you watch the Olympic Games, you see each contestant waiting with eyes closed, concentrating on the mental rehearsal of going down that hill. I have done it myself before a musical performance. As I wait for my entrance, I visualize myself playing...see the notes on the page, feel the strings beneath my fingers, and hear the sound of my bow. When I do this, I play better than when I don't.

Another way to do active visualization is to set up the scene in detail, but leave out critical parts. My sister has a fear of needles. We constructed a visualization for her to do when she has to have blood drawn. She goes to a forest...a real place where she has had some happy times. In the forest there is a place to lie down and rest. She hears the wind in the trees, feels the light touch of the pine needles beneath her hand, and then she imagines someone there who is going to help her. Sometimes it is a child who comes to hold her hand. Other times it might be a good friend who talks to her in a comforting manner. It's not always the same, but it always works. The lab people no longer turn pale when they see her coming. In fact, she was recently placed on insulin therapy, and is giving herself injections with no trouble.

Five Steps to Effective Visualization

1. Be comfortable. Wear clothing that is loose and soft. Lie down on your bed or reclining chair and allow your eyes to close when they are ready.
2. Move your arms and legs about until they are comfortable. Check for tense spots and tell those spots to relax.
3. With your eyes closed, picture furnishings in the room. Then let your mind create images of places you have been: see the trees, feel the warmth of the sun, listen to the sound of wind in the leaves, taste a wild strawberry. As you do this, it will be interesting to find newly created images creeping in, places, people and sensations you didn't expect to find. Let them all in.

4. Talk to yourself about your ability to achieve a completely relaxed state. Use affirmative, positive statements such as "I am relaxed and calm" or "I am letting go of tension" or "I am in a tranquil state."

5. Practice. For the first week, visualize briefly every hour. Set yourself up for the day by visualizing before you get out of bed or while in the shower. You will quickly find that you can visualize any time you feel the need for a tranquil state. You probably do your share of waiting...waiting for the doctor, waiting in a check-out line, waiting for a meeting to start. Visualization is particularly useful if you are waiting to undergo a medical procedure. It's a powerful tranquilizer in the dentist's chair, too.

Basic Visualization Techniques

Eye Relaxation

Close your eyes and put the palms of your hands over your eyes. Cup your hands slightly to avoid pressure on your eyelids. See the color black. Other images will intrude, but just focus on the black. You might think of a blank TV screen, a blackboard, or a piece of black velvet. Do this for two or three minutes, then remove your hands and open your eyes. Enjoy the feeling of relaxation in your eye muscles.

Metaphorical Images

Relax on your bed or comfortable chair and let your eyes close. Think about words, objects, smells, and sounds that create an image of tension. You respond with tension to things that have meaning for you. Your images will be different from someone else's. Some tension-producing images for me include a dripping faucet, an out-of-tune stringed instrument, dogs barking at night, horns honking, hospital smells, hard-rock music. Now you make your mental list.

During visualization, these tension-producing images can fade or be changed into something calming. For example, my dripping faucet fades away, no longer demanding my attention. The out-of-tune instrument can become perfectly harmonious and pleasant to hear; the barking dogs become my friends, protecting me from intruders; horns honking turn into French taxi horns, and I can imagine I'm in Paris. Hospital smells can dissipate into the air and the hard-rock music will grow soft enough to be a thunderstorm threatening in the distance.

Try this technique for tense muscles. If the muscles in the calves of your legs are tense and threatening to cramp, visualize a rope tied tightly around your legs. Then visualize the fibers of the rope separating, breaking, falling away, allowing your legs to let go and relax. Say an affirmation such as "I can let go and relax completely."

Finding Your Special Place

Everyone needs a private place. It needs to be a place where no one else can go unless you want them there. Your private place can be anywhere that is pleasant and safe, and where you feel good. You can put flowers in it, or leave it blank. You can furnish it, or leave it plain. It's your place — do with it as you will. The entrance to your place cannot be found by other people — it is known only to you. One woman created her special place as a replica of a rose garden she saw in Portland. Another created a fairy tale place with elegant furnishings and soft, pale colors. When she is in that place, she wears a floating, gossamer gown. Here is one way to get to your special, private place. You may wish to tape this and play it when you are ready for this experience. When taping, read slowly, pausing for breath. Linger on words that are especially evocative.

> Lie down or recline in a comfortable chair. Let your eyes close. Clear your mind…let it be blank and ready to receive. As you walk slowly along a country road, be aware of where you are. What is the road like?…What lies on either side of the road?…What do you see in the distance ahead?…As you progress further along the road, you see the way to get into your special place. What do you hear?…smell?…Reach out and touch the entrance to your special place.…Now you can enter this place that is private. No one can come here unless you invite them.

> Look around. What is here? Listen…Walk around…Touch things. Move things around until you are satisfied that it is a perfect place. Make yourself comfortable…Be at peace…Tranquil…Calm.

> Take your time. Memorize this place…It will always be here for you…You can come back at any time. When you are ready to leave, you go out the same way you came in…Tell yourself, "I can be safe and happy in this place. I can come here alone, or I can bring another person if I choose to do so."

> Now, open your eyes…Enjoy your tranquility…Go on with your day's tasks, completely relaxed.

The Inner Guide

You have an inner guide already, but you may not be aware of this presence within yourself. Your inner guide dwells within you and can be useful if you will listen. For some, the inner guide is a beloved person, such as a deceased parent or other special person. For some it is another self — that other you that talks to you when you're thinking. For others, the inner guide is a spiritual presence. If you wish, you may invite this inner guide to accompany you into your special place. The next time you go there simply look for your guide along the way and offer an invitation to accompany you. You will have no difficulty in recognizing your guide — you will feel right with your guide. Your guide may have an unexpected appearance, or may not take a visible form, but you will still know when your true guide is there. If another appears who does not seem right, simply send it away. Once you and your guide are together in your special place, you can let your guide know of special concerns you may have. Then listen. The answer you receive might be words, a look, or an impression.

Affirm for yourself that you are safe in your special place. Say, "I am tranquil here. I can relax completely."

Music

Many people use music to relax. Some people use music that doesn't sound at all relaxing to me, but those people probably don't like my kind of music either. Choose music that has a soothing effect for you. If this idea is new to you, go to the library and check out tapes of many different kinds of music. There are books about using music for relaxation and healing, but trial and error is a good way to find out what you want. There is sound evidence that music from the baroque period is most compatible with biological rhythms. Baroque music includes Bach, Handel, Haydn, Scarlatti, Vivaldi, and others. The rhythms in this music are regular and predictable...like your heartbeat and your breathing.

A half-hour of appropriate music in a quiet place, where you will not be interrupted, can ease tension and pain and help you to relax. Use affirmative statements at the beginning and end, such as "Music relaxes me" or "I am harmonious with the universe."

Frances

Frances is 68 years old. She and her husband care for her parents, who are in their 90s. Every day is a new crisis. One or the other of the parents is always getting sick, falling down, or needing some kind of right-now attention. Frances was in good health before her parents moved in, but now she has headaches, muscle spasms in her back, and constant feelings of anxiety. Some days she wonders how she can face another day. No matter what she does, it isn't quite right because the elderly parents are set in their ways. Frances can never do anything the way they would have done it. One or the other of them is usually a little mad at Frances. Frances is usually a little mad at her husband, since it wouldn't do to be mad at the old people.

"Don't take it out on me," Don said, "If you're going to be mad, be mad at the people you're really mad at."

"I can't be mad at my parents...they're like children," Frances said. "But I think I can get into a better frame of mind if you take them out for an hour. I need to work on myself."

On Sunday afternoon, Don took his parents-in-law out for a drive. Frances took the phone off the hook and went into her bedroom to lie down. Although she didn't have a specific plan, she decided to trust her mind and try a passive visualization. She closed her eyes and relaxed in the way she had learned with autogenic training. Then she began to visualize images for tension. She saw her father spilling cranberry sauce on the good white tablecloth. She heard her mother and father bickering over what TV program to watch. She smelled the faint odor of urine emanating from her father's clothes.

Then Frances began to let these images change. She saw the cranberry stain dissolving and disappearing in the washing machine. She heard her parents' bickering begin to sound like small children at play, and she sensed the urine smell change to the sunshine aroma of line-dried diapers. A peaceful feeling crept over her.

Finally, Frances scanned her body for tension. She recognized the feeling of strain and tension in her back and visualized a pitchfork being thrust into her flesh. At that point she was able to imagine the pitchfork softening and turning into warm hands massaging away the tension. She said to herself, "I can relax anytime I want to," and then she repeated the word "Tranquil."

When Don and her parents came home, they found a relaxed and smiling Frances. Her father noted with approval the plastic tablecloth, and her mother spoke softly.

"My tension was responsible for some of their behaviors," she told Don. "I'm not going to let it build up like that again."

Take time now to create a visualization. Find a quiet place where you will not be interrupted and follow these steps:

1. Make yourself comfortable on your bed or reclining chair, using pillows as needed. Let your eyes close as they will.
2. Monitor your body for tension. If you find a muscle or an arm or leg that feels tense, tell it to let go…relax. Then say the word "Tranquil."
3. Picture a place where you have felt peace. It may be a place where you've been, or a place where you'd like to go. Let yourself be there…feel the peace…hear the sounds of that place…let your senses fully experience that place.
4. Allow your deeper mind to direct your thoughts to a problem you have been struggling with, either now or in the past. Several images may present themselves, but the most urgent one will appear stonger and clearer than the others.
5. Now talk…talk to your inner guide, or to yourself…you know what feels right. Explain your feelings and concerns, and ask for guidance. Then *listen*. Stay focused and open, ready to receive guidance.
6. Say an affirmation of your own making. It could be something like "I am peaceful and in control of my life," or "I have a comforter and a guide."
7. When you feel that your problem is solved and you are content, open your eyes, take time to orient your surroundings, and then go on with your day.

Visualization and Behavior

Visualization can also be used for *rehearsing* behavior. If you know you have a tough situation coming up, you can prepare by visualizing the situation the way you want it to be. It's something like using a computer. You type in a paragraph and it doesn't express what you really meant, so you just backspace until it's gone and then you try again. That's a rehearsal. It's a trial-and-error process. Suppose you have been invited to give a talk on water conservation to the garden club. You feel anxious about it because you are not an expert, and you worry that the audience will not accept you. The more you think about it, the worse you feel. Your stomach churns, you can't concentrate on anything, and you can't sleep. Using the techniques described above, you can both calm yourself and prepare to perform with confidence.

For instance, you might picture yourself in your special place, recovering a familiar feeling of calm. Instead of staying there throughout the visualization, you might have your guide lead you out to the garden club. The important point is to see yourself performing successfully. Visualize the people as friendly and interested. Hear them saying that they need information on water conservation because they don't know very much about it. Smell the flowers that have been brought for a demonstration. See yourself nicely dressed, looking your best. Listen to the applause, and feel the strength in your legs as you walk back to your seat. Feel the blush of success and see the happy smile forming on your face. Once you've walked yourself through such a successful performance, you can only anticipate further success.

When you are satisfied with your visualization and you feel good, open your eyes and stretch. The following example demonstrates the true power a convincing visualization can have.

Bertha

For many years, Bertha had struggled with systemic lupus, an autoimmune disease. Now she was in the hospital because the disease was affecting her kidneys. While she was waiting for the tests, she went downstairs to the medical library and studied up on lupus. She saw how antibodies were binding to her own cells and circulating in clumps too large to be filtered by the kidneys. It sounded like she was going to have to take some pretty high-powered drugs, and she didn't like the sound of the side effects.

Back in her room, Bertha sat by the window looking at a mountain peak in the distance. I'm only 63, she thought, I can't just give up. She climbed into bed and arranged herself for her deep breathing exercises. This made her feel better, calmer, more able to think, so she decided to create a visualization.

Bertha saw the immune complexes that were causing all the trouble. "Now see here," she said to one cell group, "what you're doing is unacceptable. I don't like it, and I want you to unglue yourselves from each other. Let go. Leave me alone." It seemed she needed some solvent, so she visualized a faucet, turned it on, and filled a cup with special antibody solvent. Pouring it over the nearest group of clumping cells, she was pleased to hear the sound of something fizzing, like the sound of snow sliding off the roof. She immediately felt a warm, peaceful feeling and drifted off to sleep.

Two days later the doctor came to tell her the results of her tests. "It's not quite as bad as we thought. We can probably continue with a conservative treatment. We need to keep a close eye on you, though, in case things get worse."

Bertha smiled. That was what she had expected. She had felt a change in her body during the visualization, but she didn't feel like sharing that with the doctor. I don't think he'd understand, she thought, I'll just keep doing it and see what happens.

At the present time there is no way to prove that there were physical changes as a result of Bertha's visualization. Actually, there is a way, but no one wants to do it. You would have to have 50 lupus patients with identical signs, symptoms, and serology. Then you would give them a battery of tests, have them do the same visualization in the same way, and test them again. You would have to do this again and again over a long period of time. While this is going on, there would be another 50 patients who were like the first 50 in every way, and who would receive the same medical treatment but without visualization. It's nonsense, of course. If you do a visualization and get better, that's all that matters. A visualization is private, a personal creation that won't do for anyone but you. It comes from within your mind with it's great storehouse of experience and knowledge. It's your inner wisdom. It's powerful. Use it.

For Life

All of the techniques described in this chapter have been demonstrated to be successful in helping people obtain peace, take control over their lives, and generally remain in a better state of health. Some techniques will work well for you, some not as well. Try them out. Then work the best ones into your daily routine. Going through complete natural breathing, autogenic training, and visualization as a regularly scheduled part of your day will keep you in shape to handle the sorrows, trials, and challenges that come your way. This is the same as brushing your teeth — you do it every day for the rest of your life.

You have much more control over your "self" than you imagine. The skills you've learned in this chapter will help you to have even more control. Your life can be better, but it's all up to you. Here's something by an anonymous philosopher that inspires me when my motivation is weak.

> You are the fellow that has to decide
> Whether you'll do it or toss it aside;
> You are the fellow who makes up your mind
> Whether you'll lead or linger behind,
> Whether you'll try for a goal that's afar
> Or be contented to stay where you are.
> You can take it or leave it, here's something to do,
> Just think it over, it's all up to you.
>
> Anon.

References

Besant, A. (1976) *An Introduction to Yoga.* 10th ed. Aydar, Madras, India: The Theosophical Publishing House.

Christensen, A., and D. Rankin (1979) *Easy Does It Yoga for Older People.* New York: Harper and Row.

Cousins, N. (1980) *Anatomy of an Illness.* Boston: G.K. Hall.

Davis, M., E.R. Eshelman, and M. McKay (1988) *The Relaxation & Stress Reduction Workbook.* Oakland, CA: New Harbinger Publications, Inc.

Evan, R. (1971) *Richard Evans Quote Book.* Salt Lake City: Publishers Press.

Fanning, P. (1988) *Visualization for Change.* Oakland, CA: New Harbinger Publications, Inc.

Feldenkrais, M. (1977) *Awareness Through Movement.* New York: Harper and Row.

Hittleman, R. (1983) *Yoga for Health.* New York: Balantine Books.

Jencks, B. (1973) *Exercise Manual for J.H. Schultz's Standard Autogenic Training and Special Formulas.* Salt Lake City: private printing.

Kent, H. (1980) *A Color Guide to Yoga.* Maidenhead, England: International Book Productions, Berkshire House.

Pelletier, K.R. (1977) *Mind as Healer, Mind as Slayer.* New York: Dell Publishing Co.

Selye, H. (1950) *Stress.* Montreal: Acta, Inc.

Vithoulkas, G. (1980 *The Science of Homeopathy.* New York: Grove Press.

7

The Challenge of Illness

The other day when I stopped by a doctor's office to leave some papers, I noticed a letter taped to the wall. Written in a child's scrawl, and nicely illustrated in red crayon, the letter said, "You're a good doctor, but being sick is the pits." That sums it up no matter your age. No one likes to be sick. The scary thing for older people is that an illness that is mild in a young person may be a complicated affair when you're over 60.

Then there is the problem of getting prescriptions and taking care of yourself when you don't even feel like getting out of bed. Just going to the doctor to receive confirmation that you are sick enough to need medicine can be a chore. You also face certain challenges that are unique because of your age.

If you can identify the challenges, give them a name, and have a plan for handling each one, illness will be less overwhelming. As in other areas of your life, you need to make decisions and be prepared while you are well. It takes strength and quite a lot of courage to cope with the complexities of the medical system. That can be trying even when you are in the best of health, and it becomes nearly impossible when you are sick.

Advance Preparation

Relationships With Your Doctors

First of all, after reading Chapter 1, you will have your Inner Systems Inventory filled out and ready to take with you when you visit the doctor. Be aware that you can get into trouble when you have too many doctors. If you have a heart doctor, a lung doctor, and an allergy doctor, and none of them know what the others are doing, your problems will be multiplied.

Audrey had a serious heart condition for which she saw a cardiologist at regular intervals. When she developed a swelling in her neck, she assumed it was a thyroid problem and took it upon herself to seek an endocrinologist. He began his evaluation, prescribed some drugs, and arranged for regular follow-up. After she developed vaginal bleeding and wasn't satisfied with what the endocrinologist said, she added a gynecologist to her list. All of these doctors were conscientious about getting records from the other doctors, but there was no one in charge of coordinating Audrey's treatment. All of these doctors were giving her drugs.

After a few months, Audrey became ill. It was a puzzling illness that didn't seem to fit any particular disorder. When it began to affect cardiac function, Audrey's cardiologist hospitalized her. Many tests were done, but a blood drug screen was not done. It was an intern who solved the mystery. As part of his training he was required to get a complete history on every patient assigned to him. Some patients resented this intensive questioning because they believed their own doctors had all the history that was needed. Fortunately, Audrey didn't mind. The intern was shocked to learn that Audrey was taking several drugs that interacted badly with each other. He talked to the doctors who had prescribed for Audrey and who were somewhat chagrined to learn that Audrey's problem was drug toxicity and drug-drug interaction.

Whose fault was that? It would be easy to blame it all on the doctors, wouldn't it? And they are to blame, but you can't overlook Audrey's role in this tragedy. In the first place, Audrey didn't consult with her cardiologist about her desire to see an endocrinologist, nor did she tell the first two that she was seeing a third doctor. In the second place, she never remembered to tell each doctor about the drugs the others had given her, and they didn't always ask. And finally, she got her drugs at two different pharmacies, so the pharmacists didn't have an accurate record of her prescriptions. It was very lucky for Audrey that the problem was solved. She recovered without serious damage. Her cardiologist put her in touch with a family practice doctor, and an agreement was made that this doctor would be kept informed of visits to other doctors, as well as what drugs were prescribed. Audrey also agreed to obtain her prescriptions from only one pharmacy. The pharmacist keeps a computerized record of Audrey's drugs so he can inform her and her doctors immediately, if her drug combinations are dangerous.

Be the One in Charge

The first step toward taking charge of your medical care is to choose one primary care doctor. This doctor can be an internist, a family practice specialist, or any other health physician who meets two requirements. First, he or she must be willing to accept responsibility for coordinating your care with other specialists. Second, he or she needs to be someone you like. It is impossible to emphasize enough the importance of having a doctor you trust, someone you feel comfortable with, an understanding person you can talk to easily. Your doctor needs to be open to your ideas about what is wrong and to what kind of treatment you need. You need to be partners. On the other hand, you need to keep an open mind about your doctor's opinions and suggestions. They may reflect technical knowledge that you don't have, but the doctor must respect the fact that you know your "self" and how your body has responded in the past to certain kinds of treatments.

One of the problems that led to Audrey's difficulty was her attitude toward doctors in general. When consulting a doctor, the dialogue went something like this:

Doctor:	Your vaginal bleeding is probably due to some dryness and atrophy of the vaginal wall, nothing serious. For now, let's just have you take a little estrogen. That'll be good for your bones, too. You get this prescription filled and come back in three weeks.
Audrey:	All right, doctor. Thank you.

After leaving the office, Audrey said to herself, "I wonder if he knows what he's doing. I guess he does. It won't hurt to take the pills, anyway." Then she dismissed it from her mind. And that is the way it went with every doctor she visited, never asking questions and never sharing any information about other prescribed treatments. Audrey felt intimidated by doctors, and had difficulty conversing with them. She was sure that whatever she said would sound ignorant, so the best plan was just to agree and do whatever the doctor said.

It's a good idea to examine your own attitudes about doctors. First, you need a way to get the kind of doctor you need. One way to do that would be to have some method for evaluating your doctor as objectively as possible. The doctor needs a report card, one that only you will ever see. Take a look at the 20 statements on the following page — the Doctor's Report Card. Circle your answers. At the end, count your "yes" answers. You should have more "yes" than "no" answers, but even after doing this evaluation, your final decision will be affected by your intuitive feelings about the doctor. This report card will be good to use when you have to choose a new doctor, too.

If, after filling out the report card on your present doctor, you feel you would like to change doctors, the following steps can help you find someone who is really better for you.

Five Steps to Finding a New Doctor

1. Talk to your friends about their doctors. Ask them the "Doctor's Report Card" questions. It would be a rare doctor who would be liked by absolutely everyone, so don't expect that. If you get more than one out of four negative reports, move on to another doctor's name.

2. Find out where the doctor went to school, how long he has been licensed, and what special certification he may have. Degrees, titles, and certificates do not make a good doctor, but knowing that a doctor had enough knowledge and dedication to get them is one factor in his favor. Certification by a specialty board is of significant importance because the doctor had to pass a rigid examination. Certificates from semi-

DOCTOR'S REPORT CARD

1. When I call my doctor with a question, I know that she will call back, even if it takes quite a while. **Yes No**

2. When I call to report back after receiving treatment, he sounds interested and willing to discuss my problem further. **Yes No**

3. If I have a problem that seems like an emergency, I am able to talk to the doctor right away. **Yes No**

4. When I go to the office and have to wait a long time, she always gives me as much time and attention as she does on days that are not so busy. **Yes No**

5. He listens when I talk. **Yes No**

6. She respects the knowledge that I have about myself. **Yes No**

7. He engages in brief social conversation. **Yes No**

8. She is willing to say, "I don't know." **Yes No**

9. He is willing to consult with specialists who may know more about my problem than he does. **Yes No**

10. She keeps track of my medications, no matter who prescribed them, and how they are affecting me. **Yes No**

11. He answers questions and refers me to printed materials that will help me understand my problems. **Yes No**

12. Her manner toward me is one of respect, recognizing that I am an intelligent person, and that my time is important. **Yes No**

13. When I am in the hospital, he takes time to explain procedures and allay my fears. **Yes No**

14. If I am overly anxious, she will talk with me rather than add another drug. **Yes No**

15. He is willing to talk to members of my family. **Yes No**

16. She is open to discussing alternative treatments. **Yes No**

17. He has my living will in my record and has agreed to honor it. We have discussed what my wishes are in case of terminal illness. **Yes No**

18. She is conservative, and chooses the least harmful course of action, saving more aggressive measures for emergency situations. **Yes No**

19. I know what his credentials are, and I believe that he is competent. **Yes No**

20. I feel comfortable with her. I would not be afraid to discuss any issue. **Yes No**

Out of these 20 statements, have you been able to answer "yes" to at least 15? Less than that would suggest that you might want to investigate having another doctor.

nars and workshops are meaningless because it is easy to get the certificate without actually mastering the material.

3. Talk to your pharmacist. This professional has to deal with doctors on a daily basis, and has unique insights into their prescribing behavior and their ability to resolve drug problems. Ethically, the pharmacist may not be able to say, "Don't go to Dr. Jones," but she can tell you, "Yes, I would feel OK about going to that doctor."

4. Talk to nurses. You probably know some, or have friends who do. The hospital nurses see doctors at their best and at their worst; they know what each doctor's attitudes is about his patients, how amiable he is to work with, and they are also in a position to observe his mistakes.

5. When you have found someone you think might be good for you, make a get-acquainted appointment. Tell the receptionist you just want to talk with the doctor about your medical history and see if the two of you can work together. It costs money, but it's worth it. It's cheaper than getting started with someone and then finding out in the middle of a crisis that you can't stand him and don't trust him. While you are there, talk to the insurance person and make sure your insurance will be accepted. Find out if the doctor accepts Medicare patients. If not, you can assume this is not the place for an older person.

Talking to Doctors

Doctor Finney's receptionist looked up to see Mrs. Green approaching the counter.

Receptionist: (*to the new insurance clerk*) Oh no, here comes the old crock.

Clerk: Why do you call her that?

Receptionist: Because she rambles on and on about her aches and pains, and you can never find out exactly what she wants to talk to the doctor about.

Clerk: You mean she doesn't really have anything wrong with her?

Receptionist: Oh no, she has a lot of problems, but she doesn't know how to ask for what she needs. You get confused trying to follow her ramblings. It's sad to say, but we all get annoyed with her at times. If she would just say, "I need my blood pressure checked," or "I think those blue pills make me sick," it would be so much easier...and more pleasant, too.

Unfortunately, this is not a made-up bit of dialogue. I have heard this one and others like it many times. I'll tell you what the problem is. It's hard to know what signs and symptoms are *important* to tell a doctor, so you tell everything you can think of. I've done it myself. This confuses the doctor, wastes time, and interferes with efficient diagnosis and treatment. You go away dissatisfied because your complaints were not properly attended to, and that is the beginning of a vicious cycle. When you feel that the doctor has not understood your problem, you look for more things to tell, hoping to make things clear. Now you've added to your list of complaints, which adds to the doctor's confusion, which aggravates your dissatisfaction and frustration, and around you go again. Do you see that there are two problems?

The first problem is that you need to know how to talk to the doctor, and the second problem is that you need to know that you are heard. If you learn how to talk to the doctor, you'll find that his hearing will improve remarkably. There are several rules for talking to the doctor about a problem.

Three Rules for Talking to Doctors

Rule 1: Be Prepared

The first part of a visit to the doctor involves preparation. Before you go to the doctor's office:

- Write down all of your questions. After you've written as many as you can think of, limit the list by cutting out any redundancies. Then decide which questions are truly important. It can help to assign numbers to each — you may only decide to ask the five most important questions.
- Write out a list of all the medications you are taking and all other doctors you have been seeing. You will give this list to the doctor. He may also want to see the bottles, so bring them along.
- Think about what makes the problem feel better and what makes it feel worse. Also determine the times of the day when it acts up. Write these in your notes.
- Arrange for a friend or family member to accompany you to the doctor's office. Two heads are better than one. You will want someone to compare notes and information with after the consultation. If this is not possible, bring a tape recorder along.

Rule 2: Active Listening

Once at the doctor's office, allow the doctor to control the first part of the conversation. You can help this part move swiftly and efficiently by following these guidelines:

- State your problem in one sentence, such as "I have a pain in my abdomen." That's all she needs...more will confuse her at this point.
- Wait and listen for questions. Give your total attention to the question. You won't understand the question if you're busy formulating an answer. Wait until the question is ended before making a reply. If you're not sure what was wanted, say, "I didn't understand the question."
- Answer only what was asked. Adding other comments at this point will only cloud the picture.

- If asked, "Where does it hurt?" point to the spot and say, "Here." There is no need to add, "But sometimes I have pain in my leg, too." Eventually, the doctor will say, "Do you have pain anywhere else," or "Is there anything else I need to know?" Wait for the question. It's kind of like a tax audit. The examiner doesn't know what to do with a statement like this: "Yes, that was our income for 1987, but back in 1943 we sold a house for a loss, and then in 1989 we bought it back again and paid way too much money, but that was because my brother Harry was sick and needed a place to live, so our income in 1990 isn't representative of our true state." I can't even make sense out of that and I wrote it.
- When asked to describe pain, use words such as these: burning, stabbing, aching, or throbbing. Choose *one* word that best describes what you feel.
- Bite your tongue and refrain from saying "It's awful" or "I can't stand it" or "It's the worst pain I've ever had in my life." Avoid exaggerated statements...*crocks* use exaggerated statements. Instead, quantify the pain on a scale of 1 to 10, with 1 representing mild pain and 10 representing very severe pain. Try to be as objective and honest in this appraisal as you can.
- Use your notes to decribe what makes it feel better and what makes it feel worse.
- Give the doctor the list of drugs you are taking and the names and addresses of other doctors who have treated you. Tell what each doctor did for you. (Smile and act friendly. Above all, be honest.)

Rule 3: Ask Questions

At some point, you will be given an opportunity to ask questions. If the doctor hasn't offered you this opportunity and the discussion seems to be ending, tell the doctor you have prepared a few questions. The doctor will certainly allow them.

- When you ask a question, listen to the answer. Repeat back what you heard, to make sure you have understood. If you did not understand, tell the doctor.
- Write down the doctor's answers. Record the doctor's exact words, or your own words that the doctor has said "That's right" to. These notes will be valuable after the session.
- If the doctor has recommended surgery or any other radical treatment, ask what other options exist.

Remember that there are always options. Sometimes doctors talk as if there is only one answer to a problem. That is rarely ever the case. You can get a second opinion, and you can do some research on your own. Explore the possibilities before consenting to any treatment or surgery about which you feel uneasy. By the time you have done all this, you will probably be able to make a decision and live with it comfortably.

The next section of this chapter is designed to give you an overview of the many health care options available to you. The list of nontraditional treatments is not intended as a substitute for traditional care; in fact, many of the treatments work best as adjuncts to orthodox, or allopathic, treatment. But the list is intended to remind you that there are several answers to most problems. Understanding the options and the language can help you make the best possible decisions.

Treatment Options

While the predominant health care system in the United States is orthodox, or allopathic, medicine, there are other options to explore when allopathic treatment is not enough. Allopathy seeks to create a condition opposite of disease by suppressing symptoms or destroying disease-causing organisms. If your doctor is an orthodox M.D., then you are receiving allopathic treatment. This method has advantages and disadvantages, and sometimes another form of treatment can be helpful when the allopathic approach is weak. One major alternative approach is homeopathic medicine, described below. Following the discussion of allopathy and homeopathy is an alphabetical glossary of non-traditional treatment approaches offered for your information and exploration. These methods are generally used in addition to allopathic treatment, and they are most useful when your allopathic physician is informed about what you want to do.

Allopathic Medicine

Advantages

- Allopathic medical care is readily available in most towns and cities in the United States.
- Medical insurance, including Medicare, covers most allopathic treatment.
- Medicare is exclusively geared to this orthodox form of treatment.
- Technology exists to accomplish dramatic things, such as heart transplants, joint replacement, and other marvels. Emergency room medicine has achieved the ability to save lives in situations that were hopeless 10 years ago.

Disadvantages

- Allopathic medicine is expensive.
- The drug industry is immense, and wields power over the purveyors of the drugs.
- Medical research is astronomically expensive, and those costs are borne by you.
- Drugs have "side effects," which are actually disease states caused by the drugs. Some of them are very serious.
- Many drugs can weaken the body's ability to heal itself.

Homeopathy

Homeopathy is complimentary to other systems of health, including allopathic medicine. The word comes from the Greek *homoios* (like) and *pathos* (suffering). Homeopathic medicines seek to support the body's own defense mechanism as it becomes weakened by illness. It is a system of medicine that uses natural remedies made from animal, vegetable, and mineral substances. These are prepared in such a way that they are completely safe, and never cause side effects.

Homeopathic medicine is prescribed according to the law of similars, a centuries-old principle that recognizes the body's ability to heal itself. The law of similars states that a disease can be cured by treatment with a substance that will cause the same symptoms in a well person. A simple example would be a bee sting. The venom from the bee can cause localized redness, swelling, and pain, or it can have worse effects that may be life-threatening. A homeopathic remedy made from the essence of the bee would stop a bee sting reaction in less than a minute. Allergies are one of the areas where homeopathy has proved more effective than allopathy. The preparation of the homeopathic remedy is scientifically and rigidly controlled. Remedies have been proven through double-blind methods and have remained effective and reliable for over 200 years. Homeopathic physicians have had the same training as allopathic doctors, plus postgraduate courses in homeopathy. Homeopathy can be an adjunct to allopathic medicine and at times an alternative when allopathy fails.

Advantages

- Homeopathic remedies are inexpensive compared to allopathic drugs.
- Fewer visits to the doctor's office are required.
- The companies that produce remedies do not spend as much on research and marketing as allopathic pharmaceutical companies. There is research on new remedies, but most remedies still come from the standard repertory.
- Homeopathic remedies never cause side effects. If it is the right remedy, you get better. If it is the wrong remedy, nothing happens.

Disadvantages

- Homeopathic remedies are not covered by Medicare. Since most homeopaths have also received orthodox medical training, some insurance companies will pay for this form of treatment.
- There are not as many doctors specializing in homeopathy as there are traditional doctors, meaning there may not be one in your area. If there is, apply the Doctor's Report Card test just as you would with any doctor. Make sure the doctor has a degree in osteopathic or allopathic medicine.
- You will still need allopathic treatment at times. If you have a surgical emergency, such as a ruptured appendix, you need a surgeon.

Acupuncture

One of the oldest systems of medicine in the world, acupuncture has been practiced in China for at least 5,000 years. Therapy consists of inserting very fine needles into specific sites (365 in all) on the body. Often, more than one site is used because of reciprocal connections between them. Chinese acupuncturists believe this treatment relieves pain, treats disease, and restores the balance of energy. Since it acts on the person's vital force, it is parallel to homeopathy and therefore should not be used at the same time as homeopathy. Orthodox allopathic practitioners are interested in it as a pain control technique, but it actually has a much broader scope.

Advantages

- No drugs are used.
- When used for pain control as part of orthodox treatment, some insurance companies will pay.
- There are no side effects, as there are with allopathic drugs.

Disadvantages

- A full course of treatment can be expensive.
- Acupuncture is not available in every area.
- Some practitioners call themselves fully trained, having simply taken one or two workshops. Acupuncture, when properly used, is a complicated affair. You need to check out the practitioner's training.

Alexander Technique

This is a therapy that aims to correct structural malposition of the body. The purpose is to get rid of bad habits of posture, which damage health by creating muscular and skeletal tensions. Many musicians turn to Alexander therapy for help with the problems resulting from their abnormal playing positions. It is a gentle therapy, very comfortable for older people, and completely compatible with other forms of treatment.

Advantages

- No harm can come from it; you remain in charge of your own body.
- No drugs are used.
- The movements involved are particularly gentle.

Disadvantage

- There may not be a practitioner in your area, although some physical therapists use the Alexander technique.

Chiropractic

Today's chiropractors must have four years of chiropractic college, plus two years of pre-chiropractic education. Their studies include the basic sciences, plus anatomy, physiology, bacteriology, pathology, diagnostic techniques, x-ray, toxicology, and other study areas similar to those required in allopathic and osteopathic medical schools. Students have to pass a state chiropractic board examination and complete a 600-hour externship before receiving a license to practice.

The chiropractic premise is that every body function, every organ, and even every cell is controlled by the brain. No one could quarrel with that. Since the brain stores information and sends messages to all parts of the body, chiropractic focuses on helping the transfer of these messages, which tell your body how to work, to stay healthy. If the chiropractor believes that your health problem might be due to an interruption between your brain and the affected part of the body, he will give you a series of spinal adjustments. When the spine is in proper alignment, the brain messages can travel freely throughout your body, producing a state of health.

A doctor of chiropractic has had training in biochemistry and understands the application of foods and food supplements in the care of disease.

Advantages

- Some insurances cover chiropractic, although many do not.
- No drugs are used, thus the possibility of compounding your problem with drug side effects is reduced.
- Chiropractic is somewhat less expensive than orthodox allopathic medicine.
- Use of nutrition, exercise, and sensible practices of living helps you to maintain an active part in health management.

Disadvantages

- Chiropractic may not be covered by your insurance.
- A chiropractor cannot prescribe drugs or do surgery, although many use homeopathic remedies.
- Like homeopathy, chiropractic is complimentary to allopathic medicine.

Herbalism

Because some homeopathic remedies are made from herbs, people often get confused between the terms homeopathic medicine and herbal infusion. The difference is that homeopathic medicines are taken in very dilute form and small doses, while herbal infusions are often taken in large amounts. In general, herbalists are allopathic in their thinking. They aim to suppress symptoms and don't think of the symptom as evidence of the body's effort to heal as homeopaths do.

Advantages

- As practiced by Chinese methods of diagnosis, herbalism is effective and safe.

Disadvantages

- Herbs can be dangerous. Foxglove, for example, is the plant from which digitalis is derived, a drug commonly used by allopathic physicians for cardiac ailments. An overdose can be fatal. Prescribing herbal remedies belongs only in the hands of those who are well schooled in the pharmacology of these substances.

Hypnotherapy

Hypnosis, particularly self-hypnosis, is frequently a part of the treatment regimen used by medically qualified practitioners. It is useful in pain control, controlling addictions, and restructuring negative thought patterns. Physiologic changes can be produced with hypnosis, such as raising or lowering blood pressure, and certain endocrinologic balances. It is strictly an adjunctive therapy, and should not be considered as a replacement for other appropriate care.

Advantages

- No drugs are used. In fact, hypnosis can take the place of pain killing and tranquilizing drugs.
- It is safe. No one can make you do something you don't want to do, such as commit a crime or other act that conflicts with your values and ethics.
- It is accepted worldwide as a legitimate therapy.

Disadvantages

- In the case of biochemical depression, serious mental illness such as schizophrenia, and severe eating disorders such as bulimia or anorexia, medical treatment is needed in addition to hypnosis.
- Just as you can get a bad doctor, or a bad therapist of any kind, it is possible to get a poorly trained or unethical hypnotherapist. Ask questions, check credentials, and if things don't seem right after you start...stop.

Naturopathy

A naturopath believes that the cause of illness is an accumulation of poisonous wastes in the body. In order to clear the body of these wastes, the practitioner uses a combination of fasting, colonic irrigation and enemas, followed by proper diet. A regimen of vitamin and mineral supplements is used to counteract the bad effects of years of careless eating habits.

Advantages

- No drugs are used.

- The patient is taught to follow a high-fiber, low-fat diet, preferably vegetarian. The advantages of such a diet are well supported by recent statements made by Dr. Louis Sullivan, Secretary of Health and Human Services.

Disadvantages

- Naturopaths often have no medical training. Some receive their diplomas through the mail.
- Injudicious use of colonic irrigations and enemas can do a great deal of harm. This is not to say that these things could never be helpful under certain circumstances, but you should check with your primary care doctor before agreeing to such treatment. Be sure to question the qualifications of those who wish to administer them.

Nutribionics

Bionics is a term coined by medical engineers to describe replacement of body parts with artificial parts, such as a hand, leg, breast, or even the transplantation of a kidney, spleen, or lung. Nutribionics is regeneration and repair of cells in the body. It could be thought of as "nature's surgery"...the replacement of molecular "parts." The attitude of the nutribionics practitioner is homeopathic in that the body's defense mechanisms can be stimulated to produce healing on its own through the use of nondrug substances made from animal, vegetable, and mineral sources. Homeopathic remedies may be used. Careful attention is paid to stresses in the person's life and to environmental factors that may affect health. A diet of fresh fruits and vegetables and of whole grains is recommended. The treatment program for each person is tailored specifically for that person and takes into consideration the physical, emotional, mental, and spiritual statuses. The nutribionics approach was developed over the past 15 years at Biochem Research by its president, biochemist Dr. Horton Edgar Hodsen. Nutribionics is the service mark of Biochem Research. Still unproven by traditional scientific methods and standards, nutribionics has a good track record for healing in cases where allopathy has failed.

Advantages

- No allopathic drugs are used. Consequently, there are no drug-induced illnesses.
- Cost is less than for orthodox medical treatment.
- Each person is evaluated as a person, not a disease. Symptoms are important as indicators of the strength or weakness of the defense system. Therefore, treatment does not suppress symptoms; it supports the system so that it can heal. When healing occurs, symptoms diminish.
- It is complimentary to other medical care. Consultations with other practitioners are sought as needed.

- Rather than practicing the hands-on "art of medicine," it is a computerized service available everywhere in the world.

Disadvantages

- Nutribionics is a new field. The person who plans your program will be a voice on the telephone — Hodsen himself — rather than a personal visit to an office. The personal visit isn't necessary, but it's a different way of doing things and may be a little hard to get used to.
- Insurance doesn't cover this kind of treatment, but you'll pay less for supplements and remedies than you do for drugs.

Occupational Therapy

Occupational therapists use many of the strengthening exercises and massage techniques that a physical therapist does. Their unique contribution, however, is in the area of teaching daily living skills. For the person who has had stroke or has severe arthritis, an occupational therapist is essential. You have a lifetime of making beds, spading gardens, and brushing your teeth which may not work for you anymore. A disability that interferes with normal activities is a lot easier to handle after you learn new ways to do them. Even tying shoes can be frustrating if your hands are gnarled and you can't bend over. There is a way to accomplish nearly every task, and an occupational therapist is the one who can figure that out. He or she has also had to receive training and must be licensed.

Advantages

- If occupational therapy has been prescribed by a physician, insurance will pay.
- This is strictly an adjunctive therapy...it works hand-in-hand with the general treatment program your doctor has prescribed for you.

Disadvantages

- There are really no disadvantages unless the occupational therapist offers advice counter to that given by your doctor. In that case, you need to ask questions, get other opinions, and decide who is right.

Osteopathy

Although osteopathic doctors have as much and very similar training as that of medical doctors, they are not considered to be allopathic. They take a more holistic view of the patient, are more conservative, and prescribe fewer drugs. Like the homeopath, osteopaths believe in the body's ability to heal itself, and like the chiropractor, they use manipulation when appropriate. In all other respects, there is no difference between a doctor of osteopathy (D.O.) and a doctor of medicine (M.D.)

Advantages

- An osteopath is more likely to take a "wait-and-see" approach before prescribing drugs.
- Osteopaths will use drugs when necessary. Some also use homeopathic remedies.
- Osteopaths are more inclined to look at the patient in the context of his or her environment.
- Because of the belief that signs and symptoms of disease may be caused by misplacement of the bones, particularly the vertebrae, an osteopath will use techniques to restore the musculoskeletal system to normal.

Disadvantages

- Cost is equivalent to allopathic treatment, but is covered by insurance and medicare.
- Osteopaths are fewer in number, although they're growing.

Physical Therapy

This is another adjunctive therapy, although you can certainly consult a physical therapist without a doctor's order. The physical therapist is interested in the alignment of the musculoskeletal framework and in diseases that affect the muscles and joints. He or she has a number of modalities with which to work, such as heat, massage, electrical stimulation, and manipulations. The physical therapist has to have been trained and then licensed in order to practice.

Advantages

- No drugs are used.
- Surgery on joints can sometimes be avoided.
- This therapy is educational in nature. You can learn to do exercises at home to correct problems and to strengthen weak muscles.
- Treatment is nearly always covered by insurance.
- It is rehabilitative.

Disadvantages

- An incompetent therapist could do damage or could worsen an existing condition, but so can an incompetent doctor. You have to make inquiries about any health care professional.

Psychotherapy

Psychotherapy can be behavior-oriented or insight-oriented. A third school of therapy, cognitive therapy, emphasizes changing the pattern of your thinking and beliefs. Psychotherapy is practiced by psychiatrists, psychologists, clinical social workers, and licensed counselors.

Of the above, only psychiatrists are medical doctors: allopathic, osteopathic, or homeopathic. These three can prescribe drugs or remedies. Psychologists cannot prescribe drugs, but are skilled in the use of psychological tests. They can assess cognitive impairments, and are often skilled in stress and anxiety reduction treatments, as well as individual and family therapy. Clinical social workers tend to see the patient more holistically, taking careful consideration of the social and environmental systems that affect how the person handles stress and illness. They might be said to be homeopathic in attitude, although they do not use either drugs or remedies. Licensed counselors are more narrowly trained, focusing on specific issues such as marriage and family. Psychotherapy is usually adjunctive to other forms of treatment.

Advantages

- It is always helpful to talk things over with someone who is skilled in communication. Many of life's problems are hard to bear alone.
- When dysfunctional behaviors are present and the person is not able to change without help, psychotherapy often provides the necessary guidance.
- A highly trained, ethical, and competent therapist can help you make changes that will improve your life dramatically.
- Treatment by licensed psychotherapists is usually covered, at least in part, by insurance.

Disadvantages

- Sometimes it is difficult to find a therapist who will provide the treatment you need. You will need to seek recommendations from your doctor or another professional person. Sometimes a friend has had good luck with a therapist and you can follow up on that recommendation. It also involves some trial and error. If you don't see any progress or you feel uneasy after four sessions, you should probably try another therapist.
- Unethical and incompetent therapists do exist, just as unethical workers in any area exist. You need to be cautious about choosing the person to whom you will reveal a great deal about yourself.
- The therapist may not know when to stop. Delving deeper than the presenting problem can create more problems.

It may be that at certain times you could benefit from the combined services of allopathic, homeopathy, chiropractic, nutribionics, and osteopathy medicine since they complement each other. In fact, the chiropractor may refer you to an allopathic physician, and the homeopathic specialist may refer you to a chiropractor, or the osteopath might recommend a nutribionics approach. Any of the above may refer you to a physical therapist or any other special therapist.

However you use the services of these providers, you still need to choose one primary care doctor. The challenge is to find someone with whom you feel comfortable enough to entrust overall supervision of your care, someone who will get acquainted with your family and will keep track of medications and treatments, no matter who else may administer them. And someone you trust to have records of everything.

There are other plans that need to be made in advance of illness. Some are directives for other people, and some have to do with your coping capabilities — how you personally will get through the ordeal of illness. The rest of this chapter offers specific suggestions for advance planning. You'll find guidelines for further research, sample documents you may need to prepare, and self-reflection exercises to bring you in touch with your fears and feelings about health care. As you may have found by now, ignorance is *not* bliss when your health is concerned.

Preparing for Hospitalization

Hospitals can represent security and salvation, or they can be symbols of pain and terror. However you feel about hospitals, you need to acknowledge the fact that almost everyone — including you — will visit a hospital at some point in life. Your chances for hospitalization increase as you grow older. By taking control now, you can avoid the unpleasantness a hospital stay can represent. You might never have to go, but you never know.

In order to plan intelligently for possible future hospitalizations, it helps to get in touch with your feelings about hospitals. Harry, for example, had bad memories of childhood illnesses. Twice he was hospitalized for a month or more. He was placed in a children's ward with extremely ill children. His mother was not allowed to stay with him. The rule was that parents could only visit at certain times of the day for half-an-hour. At age three, Harry knew nothing of the rules; he only knew that his mother had gone off and left him crying in a terrible place full of strangers.

Now, as an adult, Harry hates hospitals. He knows children are not left alone anymore, but that doesn't erase his memory. Just driving by is enough to make him feel breathless and ill at ease. Consequently, it is difficult for him to include plans for hospitalization in his preparations for the future.

Jean, on the other hand, has only had brief hospitalizations for minor matters. She received competent and kindly care, and feels that the hospital is a refuge. It is easy for her to think about what she wants done if she becomes very ill and needs to be hospitalized.

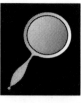

Use the following questions to help you come to terms with your feelings about hospitals.

1. I would only go to a hospital if _____
_____

2. The worst thing about hospitals is _____
_____

3. If I have to be in a hospital, I expect _____
_____

4. The last time I was in a hospital _____
_____

5. I want my family to protect me from _____
_____

6. I want my doctor to _____
_____

7. I wish the nurses would _____
_____

8. My earliest memory of being in a hospital (for myself or to see someone) is _____
_____

9. The way I feel about it right now is _____
_____

10. I might be able to handle it if _____
_____

Some of these answers will need to be shared with those around you — your family, your doctors, and possibly even an attorney. (More about legal forms and issues will follow in this chapter.) Many people play a role in a person's hospital stay, and all benefit if the patient's fears and wishes are known. By confronting these issues now, you may be able to change some of your fears. Perhaps you will decide they are not rational once you reflect on them. Or perhaps you can take action to challenge and correct your fears.

Something that has helped many people overcome fear of the hospital is volunteer work. Both men and women have enjoyed doing hospital work, reaping the reward of helping others, and at the same time becoming familiar with the workings of a hospital. There are many opportunities for volunteers. You can just about dictate what you'd like to do. Answering phones, escorting incoming patients to their rooms, and delivering flowers are common activities. Volunteers are also needed to hold babies, read to children, write letters for those too weak to write, work in the gift shop, and countless other jobs. No hospital can stay open without its volunteers. They are a valuable part of the work force.

One of the rewards is that if a time comes when you have to be hospitalized, you will not be a stranger. You already know how things are done and what to expect. You also know your way around enough to make requests and get them granted. It paves the way for your family when they have to become mediators for you in times of severe illness.

As you do advance planning for possible hospitalizations, a checklist will be helpful. Use the following as a starter, and add other items that occur to you as you go along. Once you have completed a step, put a check in the box to the right.

Hospital Checklist

1. Discuss my hospital preference with my doctor and my family.   ❑

Even though the specific hospital will be dictated by where my doctor has staff privileges, there may be choices. Doctors generally have privileges at more than one hospital.

2. Remind my family that we have as much expertise about myself as   ❑
doctors have about their specialties.

In some cases, you or your family may be the ones who know better than doctors what's right for you. Robert Mendelsohn, a pediatrician, states in his book *Confessions of a Medical Heretic* that staying close to your family is good preventive and therapeutic medicine. He says to "avoid separation whenever possible." This advice is excellent for anyone who has to be in a hospital. With the support of your family, you can become "indomitable," as Mendelsohn calls it. Stand up for what you believe and prepare your family to stand up for you. No order should be obeyed without first asking "why," and your family needs to be trained to do that. Obviously, medical personnel would prefer to have you do as you're told without question simply because it saves time and makes life easier for them. Keep in mind that they are good people, by and large, who are doing the best they can to help you. At the same time, realize that mistakes can happen and you can prevent them by questioning medications and procedures. You can do it in a way that will not sound as if you are questioning their integrity or maligning their intentions. You can let them know, by your attitude and your smile, that you are only asking for information.

3. Request that my family arrange to have someone with me most of   ❑
the time, and especially when doctors make visits.

Two heads are better than one. Sometimes when you are sick you aren't able to take in everything the doctor says. If you haven't really heard, you can't ask questions and make decisions. Your relative or friend, your "cheerleader," can be your backup ears. Then the two of you can discuss what was said, and you can make your wishes known. Your cheerleader's job is to make a nuisance of himself and make sure your decisions are honored.

Mendelsohn says that the first rule for relatives of terminally ill patients is to be immovable. If you are in intensive care, your relative should "buck the rule of the ten minute visit. Your first move should be simply to stand still. When the nurse asks you to leave, ask why. If she says your presence is too much of a strain on the patient, tell her that you are a better judge of whether your relative is strained by your presence."

Your cheerleader may not be popular with the staff, but you will get good care and your wishes will be respected.

4. Make sure my doctor places my Durable Power of Attorney or ❏
Living Will in with my hospital chart.

Discuss this document with him and with the nurses. If you can't do this, have the person named as attorney-in-fact do it for you. (Examples of these important forms are in the next section of this chapter.)

5. Have a trouble kit packed, and make sure my family knows ❏
where to find it.

Personal items make the dehumanization of the hospital bearable. Women usually know where to find the necessary shaving cream, favorite tooth brush, and other articles their husbands require, but men don't do so well. For that reason, prepare a small kit, with sample-sized toothpaste, shampoo, and so forth, that can easily be picked up and brought to the hospital. Keep it stocked and ready to go. Hospitalization is sometimes sudden and unexpected.

If you like to wear your own gowns or pajamas, you need to plan for that, also. Remember that someone is going to have to launder them, so discuss this with your family. Families are usually more than willing to take on this task, but if everyone is working and trying to schedule time at the hospital around work schedules, it may be difficult for them to take care of extra laundry. Some people have a hard time overcoming hospital depression when they have to wear the hospital gowns. In that case, it will be vitally important to make arrangements to have your own. I'm one of those people who don't care. I care about being clean, and I know I won't be wearing St. Mary's *haute couture* for long, so it's OK. My sister, on the other hand, won't stay in an ugly gown a minute longer than necessary. I'm sure she would not get well as fast if she had to wear those strange and immodest garments.

6. Have someone prepared to bring a small tape player and favorite ❏
tapes to the hospital.

Even if I'm unconscious, I want to hear music. There are certain recordings that have a healing effect on me (Borodin's second symphony, for one). Editor Norman Cousins found humor to be healing when he was ill with a rheumatologic disease, and used video tapes of comedy shows such as *Candid Camera*. Have these things ready, and prep the family so they will be able to find them easily.

7. Instruct my family as to choices of post-hospital care if I am not   ❑
able to go home directly from the hospital.

If you need a rehabilitation hospital, there may not be much choice, but if you need nursing care or just minimal assistance, there are many options, as you will see in the section on After the Hospital.

Does it seem morbid to be making plans to be hospitalized? It would be nice if you never had to go to a hospital, but the odds are that it will happen, and you might not be in control at the time. The only way you have control is to make these decisions and preparations in advance. Of course, you still want to do everything you can to stay out of the hospital. Take care of yourself!

A Living Will

The next order of business to take care of now is to decide whether you want a living will. This document states your wishes with regard to treatment and care during illness. If you feel that you do not want your life prolonged through artificial means when the prognosis for full recovery is poor, now is the time to make your wish binding. No matter how often you have expressed your wishes verbally to your doctor or to your family and no matter how strongly you all agree, those wishes can be violated. Verbal commitments have no legal strength. You need a proper document, witnessed and notarized. You can buy such a document at an office supply place, order one through the mail, or consult your attorney.

Any document you buy in office supply places in your city will be written according to the legal code in your state. As long as it is witnessed and notarized, it is a legal document, but not every state has written such documents into the law. An easy way to find out is to call an attorney's office and ask the secretary if such documents are legal in your state. You could also ask someone in the medical records department at a hospital.

Of course, such a document means that you have discussed what your wishes are with the person you name as attorney-in-fact. These discussions are not morbid. They are as interesting and important as discussing wedding plans. You didn't have any choice about how you came into the world, or what kind of treatment you would receive if you were ill as an infant or young child, but you have everything to say now about how you will be treated, and in what manner you will leave this world. The document printed here is *a sample only*, adapted from the *New York Library Desk Reference*. The form leaves room for elaboration on your personal views, but the legal essentials are here.

Keep in mind that a genuine living will is an important legal document, and a large decision to make. You may want to discuss it with your family, your attorney, or your doctor. It is for this reason you'll need witnesses before enacting your own version of this form.

Living Will

Directive to Physicians:

I,_____, of

_____,

| Street Address | Apt. No. | City | State | Zip |

being of sound mind, do hereby willfully and voluntarily make known my desire that my life not be prolonged under the following conditions, and do hereby further declare:

1. If I should, at any time have an incurable condition caused by any disease or illness, or by any accident or injury, and be determined by any two or more physicians to be in a terminal condition whereby the use or "heroic measures" or the application of life-sustaining procedures would only serve to delay the moment of my death, and where my attending physician has determined that my death is imminent whether or not such "heroic measures" or life-sustaining measures are employed, I direct that such measures and procedures be withheld or withdrawn and that I be permitted to die naturally.

2. In the event of my inability to give directions regarding the application of life-sustaining procedures or the use of "heroic measures," it is my intention that this directive shall be honored by my family and physicians as my final expression of my right to refuse medical and surgical treatment, and my acceptance of the consequences of such refusal.

3. I am mentally, emotionally, and legally competent to make this directive and I understand its import.

4. I reserve the right to revoke this directive at any time.

5. This directive shall remain in force until revoked.

IN WITNESS WHEREOF, I have hereunto set my hand and seal this _____ day of _____, 19_____.

(Signed) _____

Declaration of Witness

The declarant is personally known to me and I believe him/her to be of sound mind and emotionally and legally competent to make the herein-contained **Directive to Physicians**. I am not related to the declarant by blood or marriage, nor would I be entitled to any portion of the declarant's estate upon his/her decease, nor am I an attending physician of the declarant, nor an employee of the attending physician, nor an employee of a health care facility in which the declarant is a patient, nor a patient in a health care facility in which the declarant is a patient, nor am I a person who has any claim against any portion of the estate of the declarant upon his/her decease.

(Signed) _____
Witness

_____
Address

_____

(Signed) _____
Witness

_____
Address

_____

Durable Power of Attorney

Another way to achieve the same goal is to give durable power of attorney to someone you trust. This means that you can give another person legal power to be the decision maker in the event that you cannot speak for yourself. Here is a sample; again, you can find a legal copy of an office supply store, send for one by mail, or contact your attorney.

Power of Attorney

STATE OF _____)

) ss:

COUNTY OF _____)

KNOW YE ALL MEN BY THESE PRESENT,

That I, _____, of

_____,
    Street Address   Apt. No.   City   State   Zip

do hereby make, constitute, and appoint _____, of

_____,
    Street Address   Apt. No.   City   State   Zip

as my true and lawful Attorney-in-Fact, for me and in my name, place, and stead to:

_____

_____

I further give and grant to my said Attorney-in-Fact full power and authority to do and perform every act necessary and proper to be done in the exercise of any of the foregoing powers as fully as I might of could do if personally present, with full power of substitution and revocation, hereby ratifying and confirming all that my said Attorney-in-Fact shall lawfully do, or cause to be done by virture hereof.

This instrument may not be changed orally.

IN WITNESS WHEREOF, I have herunto set my hand and seal this _____ day of _____, 19_____.

(Signed) _____

You may want to elaborate on some of your personal views. For instance, my living will states: "1. It is my belief that death is as much a reality as birth, growth, maturity and old age; it is the one certainty of life. If the time comes when I can no longer take part in decisions for my own future, let this declaration stand as an expression of my wishes while I am still of sound mind." You can also add mention of organ donorship, or even specify how long and what kind of medications you would like to receive. Discuss these issues with your doctor or an attorney.

Once these forms are witnessed, signed, and notarized, you'll want to give a signed, notarized copy to the person you have named attorney-in-fact. Keep another notarized copy for yourself, to present to a doctor or hospital if necessary. Make sure your family knows where it is.

My sister is in precarious health, so I carry her durable power of attorney document with me, and her husband has a copy. We all rest easier knowing these issues have been considered and settled.

Managing Insurance

The next preparation you need to make is to assign someone to take care of all the insurance hassles. You need someone who will be able to plead your case to the hospital accounting department, the doctor's billing people, and the insurance companies. It is important to go over your insurance policies to determine exactly what they will cover. Armed with that information, you will be able to prepare for handling the cost of those items not covered. Filing insurance forms is sometimes an agonizing business, particularly when hospitalization is involved. There is a certain amount of work that falls to the patient. This is unfortunate unless you are prepared and have coached someone else in how to get things done. Sometimes spouses can do it, but often they are in such a state of weariness and anxiety that it is too big a task. Perhaps one of your children or a younger healthy friend could help.

Reading the insurance manuals can be confusing. Most of them have an 800 number you can call for help, but that may not be enough. It depends upon how experienced the person is who answers your call. A better source of help may be the hospital. Most have a person who specializes in insurance billing. He or she can probably help you unravel the jargon in your manual.

Identifying resources for help with insurance is an important task to do now, before you become ill, so that you can have that information listed on the cover of your manual for the person who is going to take care of things for you. You don't want to worry about this when you are lying in the hospital trying to survive.

It is best not to put things off. Spend some time with people who are most likely to be available to help you. Go over the insurance policies with them, enough so that you feel secure about how things will be taken care of. I hope you never get sick, but no one can guarantee freedom from illness. The worst thing that could happen would be a stroke or some event that would impair mental function. Since you can't predict it, you must prepare for it. Preparing now might also lift a burden of worry and denial. Your health can only profit.

Everything will be much easier if you have a record-keeping system that lists all insurance in one place. Also include bank account numbers, IRAs, and certificates of deposit. In other words, have all financial information listed in one place, with addresses and phone numbers of people to contact. The Documents Record form on the next two pages can be file-folder size, or you can have it reduced to fit into a smaller notebook. Make sure your helpers know where the form is!

Documents Record

Document	Identification Number	Where To Find	Whom To Contact: (phone/address)
Will or Trust:			
Living Will or Durable Power of Attorney:			
Medicare:			
Supplemental Health Ins.: 1.			
2.			
Checking Acct.: 1.			
2.			
3.			
4.			
Savings Acct: 1.			
2.			
3.			
4.			
IRA: 1.			
2.			

(Record continued)

Documents Record

Document	Identification Number	Where To Find	Whom To Contact: (phone/address)

CD:
  1.
 	
  2.
 	
Other Investment:
  1.
 	
  2.
 	
  3.
 	
Auto Insurance:
 	
Mortgage or Deed:
 	
Life Insurance:
  1.
 	
  2.
 	
Other Insurance:
 	
Credit Cards:
  1.
 	
  2.
 	
  3.
 	
  4.			

My copies of important documents are kept in _____ at _____
and may be obtained by _____. My attorney
is _____
_____(phone/address)_____

Money

Suppose one of the worst events does happen? Who will take care of paying bills and buying things that are necessary for your comfort and survival? Will it be the same person who handles the insurance? Most people are cautious about who has access to their money, and well they should be. On the other hand, it can be a nightmare to be incapacitated to the degree that you cannot write a check or make decisions about handling expenses.

Right now, today, you need to have someone else's name on your checking and saving accounts. The wisest course is to choose someone younger than you who is less likely to become incapacitated themselves. Very often people choose a son or daughter to be joint owners of money accounts. You know your children better than anyone. You may have one child who does not have good judgment, in which case it would be to your disadvantage to have that person accessing your accounts. The hard thing is, you will have to set aside concerns about hurt feelings and hard-heartedly choose the person most able to handle your affairs competently, and in your best interests.

Having someone else able to write checks on your account is the simplest way, but there is another alternative. Just as you have a durable power of attorney for health care, you can have one for short-term management of your financial affairs. The form is readily available at an office supply store, and you can spell out in detail how much control the other person is to have, for how long, and under what circumstances. It is a bit more complicated than the health care form, and you may wish to consult an attorney to be sure your rights are protected. Your decision about which alternative to choose is based on how much you trust the people in your life who can help you.

Amanda had never married, and it was a challenge to find the right person to carry out her directives. She had friends, of course, whom she trusted implicitly, but they were growing older, too, and couldn't be counted on to be available. It was the same problem with her brother, who was six years older than she. She finally settled on a nephew, whom she knew well, and who had proved himself to be stable and reliable in the management of his own affairs. He lived in the same city, and that was an asset, also. Amanda's lawyer advised getting a durable power of attorney, and that is what she did. She developed colon cancer a couple of years later, and all through the miserable surgeries, radiation, and chemotherapies, Amanda was relieved to have her nephew in charge. When she began to feel better, she was able to gradually resume financial responsibilities, and the nephew no longer had power. He could, of course, have power again in the future if need be.

After the Hospital

Ideally, you will return to full health after any illness or surgery and go back to your normal living situation. It sometimes happens, though, that you will not be well enough to go home. There are strict rules now about how long you can stay in an acute care hospital. If you have cataract surgery, for example, you may not go into the hospital at all, and if you do, you will be in in the morning and out in the afternoon. The only way you would stay overnight would be if you have a complicating illness, or you have some crisis arise during the surgery. Then you would likely get a new diagnosis and be allowed to stay the length of time assigned for that illness.

These rules are not all bad. They are meant to streamline the hospital process and cut costs. The trouble is that they don't fit for everyone. There are a few people who are not able to go home directly following out-patient surgery.

My friend Ned was in a weakened condition as a result of a pneumonia he had had six months previously. He just never got his strength back. His hands trembled uncontrollablly and his balance was off. It would have been dangerous for him to go home alone after eye surgery. There was the risk of falling, for one thing. With one eye covered and his balance not too good at best, his ability to ambulate was impaired. Then there were the drops to be put into his eye several times a day. Ned's hand shook too much for him to be able to do that. And what about meals? Ned was in no shape to prepare food. Of course, he wanted to go home. Ned and his family had to explore options.

He could go home with his son, but both the son and his wife worked all day, so he thought he wouldn't be that much better off. They could have a home health nurse come in to take care of the eye but that would be expensive. Ned was one year short of 65, not yet on Medicare, and his health insurance did not cover home health care. Even if they could afford to hire a home health nurse, what about meals? What about getting up in the night to go to the bathroom?

A nursing home was considered. The questions raised were: do eyedrops constitute skilled nursing care? No, anyone can do it who has clean, steady hands. Did he have any other condition which would make him eligible for a skilled care facility? No, he was just weak.

Well then, what about minimal nursing assistance, either at home or in an extended care facility? Money was a problem again. There were programs available if he had the money, or if he had none, or if he fit certain criteria. Ned seemed to fall between the cracks.

The final solution was for Ned to move in with his son for the length of time needed to build up his strength and get past the need for eyedrops. Ned's daughter-in-law arranged for Meals on Wheels for the weekdays and a neighbor to come in at intervals during the day to help Ned to the bathroom and to take care of his eye. Ned's son and his wife agreed to take turns getting up with him at night. After a month of nourishing food, Ned was strong enough to go home. The meals were continued until he was able to go out to the Gray Gourmet dinners at a nearby church.

Medicaid and Medicare

The range of services is wide, but as you can see from Ned's case, it is not always possible to gain access to them. Medicare has rigid guidelines for skilled nursing facilities. There has to be a medical condition requiring daily treatment which only a registered nurse can administer. The treatment must be such that it cannot be administered at home. These rules are always in a state of flux, and change almost monthly.

Many treatments, such as IV therapy, can be done at home now, and Medicare will pay for home health care. But again, the guidelines are rigid and inflexible, and may not fit all cases.

One step down from the skilled care facility is extended care, which is largely custodial. This is a good option when skilled nursing care is not needed, but supervision and protection are necessary. Extended care offers help with daily living tasks such as bathing, dressing, and eating. If a person cannot live at home, this is an option. Unless you qualify for Medicaid, though, money can be a problem, either because you haven't enough money or because you have too much. If you can pay $1,400 to $1,500 a month, no problem. If you can't afford that but still have more money than Medicaid allows, you're out of luck.

This is the way Medicaid works, as of this writing: if your income is below the stipulated level, a figure that is revised yearly (less than $1,221 a month now), you would be eligible for this kind of care. Included in this income figure would be interest income, veteran's benefits, annuity payments, dividends, pensions, and social security. Medicare Part B insurance premium is included as part of income.

The Asset Test for determining eligibility is given below. I think they could just call it the "acid" test. These are Colorado regulations. There may be differences in other states.

Certain resources are exempt and are not considered when attempting to qualify for Medicaid:

1. A home of any value, including the land on which it sits, and adjoining property.
2. Household goods and personal effects of any value.
3. One vehicle of any value.
4. Value of any burial space, such as gravesites, crypts, mausoleums, urns, and grave markers.
5. Value of any burial plan if it is irrevocable. If it is not irrevocable, a burial plan of $1,500.
6. Life insurance with face value of $1,500.
7. $2,000 cash.

Certain resources are considered countable and include all assets other than those mentioned above, such as cash above $2,000, other real property, promissory notes, and assets transferred to a third party within the past three years without fair consideration.

If you are married and one of you goes into a nursing home, the assets of the married couple are reviewed jointly. Exempt assets are not considered. The one who remains at home can retain half of the countable assets.

You are allowed to convert countable assets into exempt assets such as making improvements to your home or purchasing a better car and selling the old one. It isn't allowed simply to give assets away to a third party.

This is a complicated business, and you may need help. The social services office in your county is the best source of information and assistance. There are attorneys who specialize in elder law, and information may be obtained from social workers and others at nursing homes and hospitals.

Retirement Centers

Other after-the-hospital options include various kinds of retirement centers. Some of them are only for those who are entirely independent but no longer want to be responsible for cooking, cleaning, and yardwork. They range in price from $550 to $2,000 per person per month, and the decor and the services fit the price. The most elegant I've seen is very beautiful, with lovely artwork, a grand piano in the salon, and an indoor pool. Each apartment is clean and nicely appointed. A housekeeper comes daily, and a laundry service is provided. I had lunch there one day in an airy, many windowed room overlooking a sweeping lawn bordered with flowers.

Other centers I visited were of varying degrees of elegance and somewhat less expensive. The worst was a small home with only eight residents. It was not clean, smelled of fried food, and the recreation appeared to be television. The interesting thing was that the monthly fee was $600, and yet I saw another, larger center that had nice, clean rooms, good menu options, transportation, and recreation for $550. The price doesn't always tell the tale.

Two facilities had good ideas. There was a section similar to the more expensive center described above, and also a nursing home section. That means that you can live independently in your apartment, receiving some physical assistance, until you are no longer able to care for yourself, and then you can transfer into the nursing home section. The advantage is that you don't have to make an adjustment to a strange place and strange people at a time when you feel sad and disabled. Just one problem…money.

Making advance decisions about this kind of thing requires research on your part and some honest assessment of priorities. The following Retirement Center Chart will help you to make an objective evaluation of facilities you have visited. Write the name of the centers in the left-hand column, then rate each item listed across the top on a scale of 1 to 5. Use 1 for the poorest rating and 5 for the best. The center that has the most 4s and 5s will probably be the best choice. If it seems close, add all the numbers; the highest total score wins.

Living with your children was not included on the checklist because there are so many kinds of considerations influencing that choice. This option is covered in more detail in the next chapter, The Family.

Growing older also means growing wiser. Wisdom arises from the ability to think critically. Investigating alternatives and weighing options are necessary steps to making correct decisions. The decisions you make might not work at all for someone else, and what works for your neighbor could be wrong for you. The information in this book is a springboard for more learning. I hope it is opening a door for you. And I hope that what comes next will pave the way for more rewarding family interactions, too.

Retirement Center Chart

Name of Center	Cost	Location	Resident/Staff ratio	Nursing assistant	Exercise/Recreation	Accessable to visitors	Attractiveness	Friendliness/Competence of staff	Transportation	Quality of meals – Special diet	Friendliness of residents	Laundry	Housekeeping	Privacy	Grounds	TV cable hookup	Refrigerator in rooms	Microwave allowed
Example: Aspen Leaf	$1200	5	3	4	3	2	5	4	4	5	5	3	4	2	4	4	5	3

1 = poor
3 = average
5 = excellent

References

Davis, M., E.R. Eschelman, and M. McKay. (1988) *The Relaxation & Stress Reduction Workbook*. Oakland, CA: New Harbinger Publications, Inc.

Feldenkrais, M. (1977) *Awareness Through Movement*. New York: Harper and Row.

Hodsen, H. Nutribionics. Box 959, Washington, UT 84780.

Mendelsohn, R. (1979) *Confessions of a Medical Heretic*. Chicago: Warner Communications Co.

New York Public Library Desk Reference (1989). New York: Simon and Schuster.

Panos, M., and J. Heimlich. (1980) *Homeopathic Medicine at Home*. Los Angeles: J.P. Tarcher, Inc.

Richardson, S. (1988) *Homepathy, The Illustrated Guide*. New York: Harmony Books.

Vithoulkas, G. (1980) *The Science of Homeopathy*. New York: Grove Press.

8

The Family

A picture of a four-generation family is still enough of a novelty to make it into the newspaper. Last week I watched as a five-generation picture was taken. The amazing thing is not that five generations are living at the same time, but that five generations could get together to have a picture. This mobile society disadvantages families by widely separating them. Most people have a hard time getting two generations in one place long enough to take a picture. Often, when families are scattered far away, there will be nonfamily people who take on family roles. It's funny, though, that even when your family is no longer near, your life is still affected by them. One batch of statistics will say that older people have contact with some family member nearly every day, while another insists that only a few have this privilege. The truth would be hard to come by, but it doesn't matter a great deal. What matters is *your* situation, how your family relationships influence your decision making, how your decisions affect your family. As you have seen, it is imperative for you to be in charge of decisions about your life.

The plans you drew up 20 years ago probably need to be altered by new facts about your life, by the number of years you've lived, and the kinds of experiences you've had. So here you are, making new decisions. The importance of making decisions about your future cannot be overemphasized. Your ability to make decisions depends upon your ability to communicate your wishes clearly. After all, some decisions will need to be carried through by other people. The decisions have to be made now — procrastination could leave you at the mercy of someone who doesn't understand what you want. Your decision-making behavior affects the integrity of your relationships with family, and your ability to determine the future quality of your life.

This chapter has two parts. The first is written to help you consider the natural changes that take place in families over time, and work toward a new and continually fulfilling balance. The second part of the chapter is addressed directly to your adult children. If you can, share this section with them. Lend your book, xerox some pages, or just read it over yourself and discuss with them ideas that strike you. Keep in mind that no one has an "ideal" family, and you'll make yourself crazy if you imagine that every other reader has perfectly understanding children and parents. You may be considering moving in with your children, with serious reservations. You may not see this as a remote possibility. You may not have any adult children. In each of these cases, the sections that follow can offer you something. They can help you see your situation from different perspectives. They can help you understand other people's situations, and even reflect on situations from your own childhood. Somehow, a family has played and continues to play a role in shaping who you are.

Finding a New Balance

Throughout your life you have gone more or less smoothly from one role to another. This role modification is the same continuous process that you see in the lives of other creatures. I love to listen to the birds in my back yard. Even more, I like to watch them. In early spring the parents are energetic in gathering nesting materials, and then comes the egg-sitting period. Daddy bird takes his turn on the eggs so Mom can stretch her wings and get something to eat. The really hard work comes after the babies appear. The parents spend all of their time gathering food for themselves and for the babies. Eventually, of course, the babies take off on their own, and Mom and Dad get ready for the winter journey. Your life is more complicated than that, but you accomplish the role changes with about as much energy as the birds.

Sociologist Andrea Fontana points out that this continuity of changing roles is disrupted when you reach old age. There is usually a period of confusion about the new role.

Irving Rosow, another sociologist, believes there is status related to being old, but the roles are not clear. When you become old, you still retain the values and beliefs that have always guided you, but you may not have as distinct a feeling of your purpose in life. You may not know what the customary behaviors and norms are for the role of "old." These scientists suggest that this role ambiguity tends to create a condition of denial, a refusal to recognize that one is aging.

The period of transition from the role of "parent" to the role of "adult friend" to your children is rather lengthy. Once you get to that friendship period, however, you may find it to be rather brief. It may be just a few years. Soon, you start into another transition, this time moving toward more interdependence with your adult children.

This is a fluid state during which you are at times completely independent, and at other times quite dependent. This dependence is not childlike. Young children in a dependent state rarely assume responsibility for their parents. Psychologist Allan Fromme believes that in this interdependent state you never stop giving to your children. When physical capacities are diminished, the greatest gifts you give are love, interest, and the wisdom of a lifetime of experience. There are a couple of things that can happen during this time.

The lessening of your role as parent may create confusion and depression for you, or it can catapult you into a new role of your own creation. Grandparenting is one wonderful change and opportunity, and there are many more. Basically, you decide how these role changes are going to affect you. It would be best for you to decide this now.

If you do not create a new and positive role, you won't be much fun to be around. It is likely that you will either become withdrawn and depressed or you could become whiny and cantankerous. If you do decide to create a new role, aside from grandparenting, then it is likely you will be interesting, pleasant, and a joy to be around. This decision is important because it affects how other people, including your children, will treat you.

As you age, you have to face an unpleasant fact: sometimes adult children have difficulty loving their aging parents. They may go through all the motions of caring by taking responsibility for their parents' welfare, but at the same time, they are emotionally shut down. Psychotherapist Marcella Weiner and her collaborators suggest that this happens because of shock and resentment at the role reversal. When unprepared for it, adult children may feel paralyzed and unattached. When this happens, the children seldom visit their aging parents, and eventually never visit at all. This is seen too often in nursing homes. My feeling is that one parenting task you maintain forever is the responsibility to foster the new relationship you are building with your children. If you do this well, love need never be lost. Adult children who do adjust to new role changes are able to achieve even deeper intimacy with their parents. Now is the time to nurture the relationship you have with your children, help it to grow, and help them to accept the changes.

Living With Your Children

It could happen that you will decide to live with one of your children. This decision forces a confrontation with new roles and magnifies all the issues between you and your adult children. Even if you're not considering moving in, some of the issues raised here may be relevant to you. A decision to live together is made because all parties concerned truly believe it to be a desirable arrangement. It is a big step, and it can be a blessing or a curse.

In order for it to be a blessing, you will have to be harmoniously interdependent with your family as a whole. Eric Fromme likens it to musical counterpoint, and indeed that is a good analogy. A lovely Bach Fugue has four voices, each one singing sometimes alone, sometimes remaining silent, only to reenter and blend with other voices in an interwoven and harmonious whole. You need to be your own person, ordering your own life with as much privacy as can be afforded. The family needs space that cannot be violated so they can go about the business of growing and learning as an independent family. At the same time, you need to feel you are a part of this family — wanted, needed, and appreciated. They need to feel love and respect for you and from you. In this way all of you together create the harmonious whole.

Mom and Dad never stop being Mom and Dad, even when they become Grandma and Grandpa. The desire to give advice, the tendency to judge, and the yearning to change things dies hard. There are three rules which must be followed if you and your family are going to live happily together.

> **Three rules for living with your children**:
> 1. Never offer advice.
> 2. Refrain from making judgmental statements, even if they are to yourself.
> 3. Leave their house alone.

As for Rule 1, just bite your tongue. If your advice is wanted, it will be asked for.

Following Rule 2 may be difficult at times; everyone has a preferred way of doing things. Just remember that the way to be happy in your little girl's or little boy's house is to accept unconditionally everything they do and say. The one exception to this rule is if there is abuse. In that case, it is essential that you speak out. You may need to contact family members outside the immediate home, or impartial outside authorities. Look in your yellow pages under Social Services for resources.

Rule 3 reminds you that even if your children's house looks terrible to you, it's still their house. You can't change them. The only person you can change is yourself.

If you can't abide by these rules, abandon all thought of living with your children. If you can, then consider the matter of your attitude. Remember, you can't change their attitudes, only your own.

Of course, for things to move smoothly you'll want your children to follow some rules as well. These ideas will be discussed in more detail near the end of this chapter, in a section written directly for your adult children. For now, keep in mind that you never give up some basic rights and responsibilities, such as your right to privacy and to do for yourself whatever you can and want to do. The story of Tess can help you see the importance of clear rights.

Tess

Tess thought it would work out all right to live with the children. They had a nice room for her, with a place for her desk and television. She would have to share a bathroom with Sherry, her oldest granddaughter, but that surely would be no problem. Tess loved Sherry. She had resolved that she could keep the three rules, and so the move was made.

At first, if some disagreement arose between the parents and their children, Tess would just go to her room. Of course, she could see quite clearly what the parents were doing wrong, but she didn't offer advice. When she was in her room, listening to the sounds of battle, she would say to herself: "I can't judge them. They're all doing the best they can with what they know. I don't know that I could handle things any differently." The hardest thing was to refrain from trying to teach her daughter to be a more patient mother. "I can't change Angie," Tess said to herself. "I can just be patient myself."

Things went along smoothly for about three weeks until Tess and Sherry clashed over the bathroom. Sherry was inordinately long in getting ready for a date, and Tess wanted her bath so she could go to bed. After an hour and a half, Tess tapped on the door.

"Are you nearly through, dear?" she asked.

Sherry flung open the door, gave her grandmother a killing look, and stomped off into her room. Tess felt as if she had been hit.

She brooded about the incident all evening, and finally went out to speak to Angie.

"Angie, I don't know what to do. Sherry does take a long time in the bathroom, and sometimes I need to get in there. I know I've upset her, but I don't know what to do about it."

"You have to consider her age, Mom," said Angie. "You know I was the same way at that age. You just have to put up with it."

Tess retreated to her room. Angie hadn't been very interested in Tess's feelings about the matter. The more Tess thought about it, the angrier she got. "I have rights, too," she said to herself. That night she couldn't sleep. Tossing and turning, she brooded about the unfairness of Sherry's bathroom use.

The next morning Tess said at the breakfast table, "I don't think I'm wanted here; I'm going to look for a small apartment."

"Come off it, Grandma," yelled Sherry. "Quit feeling sorry for yourself."

"Well, I feel bad...," Tess began when Angie interrupted, "For Pete's sake, Mom, don't make a mountain out of a molehill."

Tess shut her mouth, and no more was said about the matter. Things were not the same in the family now. Tess was afraid to make anyone angry, and everyone else felt edgy in Tess's presence.

Communication and Rights

Problems in attitude and communication are both present here. Tess was trying so hard to obey the three rules that she forgot that she could be assertive about her own needs. She kept herself an outsider in her efforts to keep peace.

Tess needed to be clearer about everybody's rights, and to speak out appropriately in defense of them. Tess took her complaint to Angie instead of to Sherry. Her problem was not with Angie; the conflict lay between herself and Sherry. Angie was defensive and unsympathetic because she was being asked to mediate in a quarrel that wasn't hers. Sherry was hurt and angry that her grandmother had spoken to her mother. She also felt guilty about her own behavior, but she didn't have the skills to talk about it. Most importantly, no one knew exactly what their rights included, although everyone had the sense that they had been wronged.

Tess can't make Angie or Sherry happy. She can't give them communication skills. What she can do is model assertive behavior and open communication by her own actions. Negotiating rights and responsibilities for all parties is the first step.

It's best to set out rights and responsibilities for all parties as early as possible in the new living arrangement. However, it's never too late to work these issues out. By bringing them up now, Tess can undo some of the damage and hurt feelings caused by her encounter with her granddaughter. Everyone benefits from seeing their rights spelled out, and knowing that each family member cares about the other's rights.

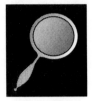 The list of rights below are those made up by Sherry, Tess, and their family. They are listed here because they include rights that many people living together agree on. You'll also see blank lines for your own additions. Take your time reading and adding to these lists. If something does not make sense to you, cross it out. The more thorough and personal these lists are, the more you guarantee mutual respect and freedom among your family members. Of course, you'll want to share your thoughts with all concerned parties, and to solicit their input. (A more generalized list of rights and responsibilities for families not living together can be found at the end of this chapter under the heading "License.")

Grandparent's rights:

- Right to privacy.
- Right to equal bathroom time. (Sherry and Tess could come to terms about specific hours for bathing.)
- Right to assistance when needed.
- Right to kitchen and refrigerator space for storing special foods.
- Right to use of the telephone, although it's better when the grandparent installs her or his own phone in her or his bedroom.
- _____
- _____
- _____

Adult children's rights: (These do not need to be spelled out in such detail because it is, after all, their home, but some are necessary.)

- Right to privacy.
- Right to time away from home alone.
- Right to help the grandparent when help is obviously needed.
- _____
- _____
- _____

Grandchildren's right: (These look a lot like grandparent's rights.)

- Right to privacy.
- Right to adequate bathroom time.
- Right to talk with grandparent alone.
- Right to talk with parents alone.
- Right to have friends if they do not infringe on grandparent's rights.

- Right to a certain amount of telephone time.
- _____
- _____
- _____

As long as you exercise your rights and responsibilities in a way that does not obstruct the rights of others in the family, it will be possible for all of you to maintain your own identities, your independence, and your special interests. You can be integrated as an interdependent group.

Even when rights are clarified, conflict will arise. That's when you'll need to rely on communication skills, such as those discussed in Chapter 4. Speaking assertively, using "I" statements, and listening actively are all essentials skills in maintaining a close family setting.

Resolving Conflict

Potential sources of conflict are food, religion, social behavior, and cleanliness. Tess solved the food problem by having a small refrigerator in the utility room in which she could keep the things she needed for her diabetic diet. This refrigerator was off-limits to the children in the home. A closet shelf in her room served to store other food items. She felt better about having some food that was just hers, rather than using the common store all the time.

If you are not all of the same religion, compromises must be made. How will you get to your place of worship? Can the family take you on the way to their church or synagogue? Perhaps you would be comfortable going with them some of the time, and they could go with you some of the time. This is where communication skills will help. It may be that you will want to ask someone in your church to take you, and avoid conflict. It sometimes happens that religion can't be discussed. If that is so, you must find ways to maintain your own religious activity, and keep your own counsel.

You are probably not used to big dinner parties, or to football orgies. If you can fit in comfortably at some of these functions and you feel welcome, don't hesitate to join in. If you find them tiring and uncomfortable, then take your supper and a special treat to your room and enjoy some solitude. Perhaps you could rent a movie you've been longing to see. You should be able to be a part of the family when it feels right, and you should be able to decline when it doesn't.

Probably more ire is raised by dirty bathtubs and hair in the sink than anything else. When you go in to have a bath after your 15-year-old grandson, you may find both, and more. What do you do? Try to clean it yourself? Call your grandson back? Snitch to his mom? How about bringing it up in a family meeting? A friend of mine swears by the benefits of regular family meetings, where troublesome issues can be raised safely, and plans and progress can be discussed. If you have a dirty tub on your agenda as a problem to be solved, the family probably has concerns on their separate agendas. Here is the way to discuss problems.

Three Steps to Discussing Problems

1. Present your concern in a pleasant, uncomplaining manner, using "I" statements. Avoid saying, "You did this," or "He always...." Say instead, "I have a problem with...," or "I feel...," or "I wonder what I can do to help...." Never resort to accusations or statements intended to make the other person feel guilty.
2. When your concern is greeted with rebuttal, look for the truth in what is said, and acknowledge it. Then continue probing for ways to solve the problem.
3. Accept suggestions and offer suggestions, going back and forth until a resolution is achieved.

Temper your independence with the understanding that from the age of 16 on, children believe they know better than their parents. So why not let them think it? If they enjoy making arrangements and taking care of you when you're healthy, then they will be prepared for doing it when you really need it. It's good training for them. As long as you are still making the vital decisions, you can relax and just revel in being part of this wonderful family you have produced.

An added attraction is that when you are called upon to tend to grandchildren, you just ask the parents for a list of rules for the children. Then, when there's a question about what they can and cannot do, you simply say, "This is what Mommy wrote down about doing homework (or practicing, or playing, and so forth)," and then you say, with a big smile and a twinkle in your eye, "and I always do what my children tell me to do." Their response will be, "Then why don't you do what we tell you?" and you can say, "Ah, but you're not grown up, yet." I have found that this ends any pleading they were planning to do, thinking that Grandma is a soft touch. It also endears you to the hearts of their parents, especially the in-law half. And this leads you into more talk about grand-children, one of the special new relationships in your evolving family.

Individual Relationships

Grandchildren

Most grandparents say that having a grandchild is like having all the good times with your own children and none of the bad. This isn't quite true, of course. When your children have trouble with their children, you suffer. The difference is that you are not directly responsible. If you're like me, you find yourself full of good suggestions about how to handle things. These suggestions are not any good (to them), of course, and they probably won't be accepted. Over the years and through making many mistakes, I have learned to *not* offer suggestions. The only way you can help is to keep your mouth shut and listen. If you are successful at this, you may find that occasionally your advice will be asked for. When my daughter, who has five children, calls and says, "I called for advice," my heart leaps with joy, and I say, "Oh good. I love to give advice." She's a smart woman. If I ever become too vigorous with my advice, she says, "Just give me your ideas, Mom, so I can think them over and make up my own mind." I appreciate these reminders because it helps me with my role transition. I need a little guidance as I let go of being in charge.

Developing relationships with grandchildren who live far away is challenging. The little ones don't make much conversation on the telephone, although it's a thrill to hear their voices. If you are having difficulty hearing, then the small high-pitched voices may be hard to understand. In order to avoid saying, "What did you say?" all the time, you may want to pretend that you have heard. That's fine with children younger than four because "Oh my!" "Really?" and "Well, well" are responses that fit most statements from that age child. When they get to be four, though, they want to ask questions and have a back-and-forth conversation, and ambiguous replies won't do. Honesty is really the best policy. "Susie, I don't hear as well as I used to. You sound very far away. I really want to hear everything you say, so could you please talk really loud for me?" It is good to repeat back to them what you think they said so they will know you are listening. For example, "Tim, I thought you said you had six new cats? Can that be right?" and then the two of you can have a good laugh when he says, "No, Grandma, I said I had a sick rat." Laughing about it lets him know that being hard of hearing is not something to be embarrassed about. Most of all, he will appreciate your interest in him.

All children like to receive letters, but not very many are good at answering. This can be discouraging. Postcards are great. Children love them, and you can write one or two messages and not feel so unrequited when there is no response. Even if all you write is, "We can see this mountain from our kitchen window" or "Sometime we'll take you to this rodeo," you are knitting a bond.

Divorce or death may produce situations in which you don't have many opportunities to see grandchildren. The new step-dad or mom may not want you to be involved in the new family life. It's harder, of course, if the grandchildren are now part of a family that does not include your son or daughter. Carol had a situation like that.

Carol

After the divorce, custody was granted to Carol's daughter-in-law, Dorina. At first Dorina didn't want to hear from Carol at all, and even wrote a letter to that effect. Carol wasn't about to be daunted in her efforts to maintain contact with her grandson, however, so she respected the letter only in part. She did not write to Dorina, but she did send cards and gifts to little Tony. Once in a while she would write a longer letter to Tony, telling him about trips she and Grandpa had taken, or about what his cousins were doing. When Tony got to be about seven, he began to call on the phone. For years Carol and Bob did not see Tony. When Tony was 12, he called and asked if he could visit. His parents had yielded to his pleadings and agreed to let him fly across the nation to see Carol and Bob. Tony said, "If it's OK, could you meet my plane?" Trying to keep the tears from running into the phone, Carol said, "Can we meet the plane? I should say we can. We'll be there with a big brass band. We're the white-haired folks wearing red hats and great big smiles."

Tense family situations are best handled with a great deal of patience. That means being available, waiting with an open heart, and biting your tongue every time you want to lash out at the unfairness of it all. There is much about life that seems unfair. By now you know that there are situations you can't fix by assertive confrontations. Some things are beyond your control and out of bounds. Why make yourself sick with anger and worry? Take nonintrusive action by writing, listening, and sending gentle reminders of your love. And all the time you wait, and wait, and wait. Everything works out eventually.

Both children and grandchildren may be involved in helping you carry out decisions. Remember that everyone has rights and responsibilities. Whenever conflict over a decision seems imminent, go through the rights and responsibilities exercises again, inserting the names of the parties involved. Do this alone at first, and then go over it with the other person if you have reached an impasse where neither of you is able to understand the other's viewpoint.

Siblings

Ideally, brothers and sisters can be seen as resources and as friends. Sometimes it's difficult to provide and receive help without drifting into dependency. Dependence upon your sister, who is also facing the challenge of aging, is not a good idea. Having your younger brother dependent upon you is not a good idea either. Here again, the rights and responsibilities exercise is a useful way to resolve dependency issues, but it only works if you are assertive, not aggressive: assertive enough to stick up for your rights without weakening your brother's rights. When you can agree to accept certain responsibilities, you are in a position to be a comfort and solace to each other. In about 70 percent of older people whom I have seen for problems concerned with decisions, siblings have been supportive, but not intrusive. Geriatric psychiatrist Alvin Goldfarb believed that dependency in old age was the result of loss. As you grow older, people leave you. They die or move away or become too involved in their own problems, and this diminishes your resources. If you aren't constantly building new resources, your losses may leave you feeling helpless and out of control. When that happens, you start looking around for help, any kind of help.

Marie

Something like that happened to my friend Marie. First her parents died, and then her dearly loved older sister. Her son and his family were transferred to Japan, and her daughters lived too far away to visit often. Of course, she could call on them, but they were of no use in an emergency. Marie had depended heavily upon her husband and never become knowledgeable about ordinary household mishaps. When her husband died, she would call her son, but after he left she didn't know where to turn. She began to rely more and more on her younger brother, to the point that she was asking for help of some kind two or three times a day. John still had teenage children at home, and he and his wife both worked, trying to support the older children who were in college. John loved Marie and wanted to help her, but the constant demands were creating stress in his family.

That's not an unusual scenario. Everyone in this family was unhappy. The son in Japan worried constantly about his mother, and struggled with indecision about whether to return to the states to be close to his mother. The daughters were not affluent, so they felt trapped and helpless that they could not take care of her. Marie was depressed and frightened, and John was dog-paddling through life trying to keep his head above water. Much of this unhappiness could have been avoided if Marie had become self-sufficient earlier in life and if she had developed new resources as familiar ones were lost. The real key to Marie's problem lay in her total dependence in the past upon her husband. It can happen the other way, too, with the husband being too dependent upon his wife.

Spouse

A couple who has lived a lifetime of 40 or more years together has an entirely different relationship from the couple who has been together only a short time. The man or woman who has had one, or at most two, marriages will have a different kind of adjustment to loss of a partner than the one who has had multiple marriages. Even with these differences, however, there are certain basic elements in the loss-dependency issue. You might look back to your Complete Living Systems Inventory from Chapter 2 to evaluate the assets and liabilities in both past and present relationships. Think about what you wrote, and check again to see if something could be added or even deleted. You need to be particularly aware of those assets and the resources they provide in helping you prevent dependency. Take time to do that before going on.

The steps you take to prevent dependency just happen to spell INDEPENDENT.

Insist upon taking part in household tasks and auto maintenance.
Never ask someone to do something for you that you can do yourself.
Develop new skills; the use of tools of all kinds.
Enroll in community classes that will help you perfect skills.
Practice what you have learned.
Exercise to stay physically fit.
Never assume things won't break.
Draw on inner strength...know that you can do what you need to do.
Engage community resources.
Nail these steps to the wall, where you can read them often.
Talk to yourself in an encouraging and positive manner.

Jacob

If you had known Jacob Weller over the years, you would never have thought he was dependent upon his wife, Erma. Jacob was a strong man and a hard worker. When he was 23 years old, he opened a hardware store with a minimal investment and no operating reserve. He made the store financially successful in about five years by doing graveyard shift at the steel mill. Those first five years were hard, and Erma had to shoulder full responsibility for running the home and bearing three children. She always said with pride that Jacob was a good provider. "We were never hungry," she said. "Jacob saw to that."

Other women in the neighborhood grew to envy Erma as Jacob's store became more and more successful. "That Jacob sure knows how to do business," they said, "he knows what to do with a dollar." What they didn't see was Erma's strength. It was Erma who paid the bills, always making sure there was something left over to put in savings. Erma was the one who took care of household repairs. When they finally had enough money to buy a car, it was Erma who kept it properly maintained. When Jacob came home from work, he found his clothes clean, his home cheerful and pleasant, and the smell of a good meal in the air. Erma made sure the children had money for college. Erma insisted that they make a will and have plans for Jacob's retirement. The one thing Erma never thought about was that she might die and leave Jacob alone. Jacob was a strong man and clever; it never occurred to her that he would feel helpless without her.

The children completed their education and became successful in far-off places. Not one was interested in the hardware store. And so Jacob went on working hard until the day he came home and found Erma dead on the kitchen floor. "Her heart just quit," the doctor said. "If she could have gotten to a hospital right away, we might have saved her...but then again, we might not. It was a bad one." The doctor told Jacob to go on and live a normal life and be glad his wife died without suffering.

After the funeral, when the children had gone and the neighbors were no longer bringing in meals, Jacob returned to the store. At the end of the day, he returned to a dark house. There was no fragrance of a meal being prepared. He went into the bedroom and sat on the edge of the unmade bed. He looked at the overflowing laundry hamper. It didn't feel like home anymore, and Jacob didn't know what to do.

Jacob literally did not know what to do. He'd never cooked a meal in his life. "Live a normal life," he said to the floor. "There's no normal life in this house anymore."

Sally

It sounds extreme, but it happens. More commonly it is the wife who has become overly dependent. Lack of knowledge of family finances is the most devastating result of overdependence for women. Sally had never had to balance a checkbook, pay a bill, or do any other normal money transaction because Bill did it all for her. He thought he was cherishing and protecting Sally. He would not willingly have admitted it, but he also feared she would not be able to learn to do it in an organized and efficient manner. There had been some verbal battles when Bill thought Sally was spending too much money, but Sally was quick to point out that she had no way of knowing the limit unless he told her. They worked it out and lived fairly amicably for 30 years.

The shock of Bill's death from cancer was greatly compounded by the overwhelming financial confusion. Since they had no children, Sally turned to her brother. He tried to teach Sally but it was difficult because Bill had an accounting system of his own design and the brother was unfamiliar with it. They managed to get through the funeral expenses and the transfer of accounts to Sally's name. There were delays, but because Bill had left a will, it was possible to make funds available for Sally's immediate use while waiting for the estate to be settled.

The whole situation made the grief process more difficult. In fact, the real work of grieving was delayed while Sally grappled with accounting procedures.

Most women are not as much in the dark as Sally was, but I have talked with a few who were. The next generation of older women will not be as helpless as this generation. Old attitudes about "woman's place" and "woman's work" are fast fading. The good that has come out of this change is that women are better able to take care of themselves. They need not be dependent on others to do the daily tasks of living. If you feel worried about your ability to fix a leaky faucet or arrange for a roofing job, don't despair. You can still learn to do these things.

Men also often find themselves overwhelmed by the tasks confronting them after the death of a spouse. Remember Jacob? After the death of Erma, he found himself ill-equipped to perform the daily housekeeping tasks so expertly performed by Erma for so many years. It doesn't have to be this way.

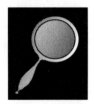

On the following page are checklists: one for women, and one for men. These lists let you reflect on your abilities and knowledge of your home environment. Answer each question by checking the box if you feel confident about the task. Then begin to learn each task, one at a time, that you could not check. If you find yourself needing help with a task, read the Resources section that follows the list. Each list contains more than a dozen elementary tasks you need to know how to do. There are others, of course, and it is up to you to expand the list as you think about things that can go wrong in your daily life.

Resources

Public library: Books on household repairs, car maintenance, and numerous pamphlets about safety, money management, and legal matters. The reference librarian can help you find what you need.

College or university: Community education classes in basic car maintenance, furniture repair, cooking, money management, and legal matters such as making a will or trust.

State agricultural college extension service: Offers many classes and pamphlet — from canning to taking care of your pet to ridding your lawn of blight. They'll talk to you over the phone about problems, too.

Rural legal aid (sometimes just called Legal Aid or Community Legal Aid): Offers some over-the-phone advice or can arrange an appointment with a lawyer for a low fee or for no fee.

As you investigate these resources, you will probably be referred to others; and the longer your list, the easier it will be to get the help you need. Other resources are also listed in the last section of this book.

Women's Checklist of Tasks

- ❑ I know where to turn off the water to the house.
- ❑ I know how to turn off the electricity.
- ❑ I know where to turn off the gas.
- ❑ I know how to replace a washer in a faucet.
- ❑ I can unstop a drain.
- ❑ I can unplug a stopped up toilet.
- ❑ I can mend a torn window screen.
- ❑ I can change a flat tire or know how to get help.
- ❑ I can add oil to the car.
- ❑ I know what needs to be done for car tune-up and other maintenance, and I know how to find a trustworthy mechanic.
- ❑ I can balance my checkbook.
- ❑ I know where important documents such as will, insurances, mortgage papers, and so forth, are kept.
- ❑ I know how to find resources and how to use them to solve problems of all kinds.

Men's Checklist of Tasks

- ❑ I know how to iron a shirt.
- ❑ I know how to sew on buttons and mend open seams.
- ❑ I can use the sewing machine.
- ❑ I can prepare all of the foods I am accustomed to having.
- ❑ I know where to find things in the kitchen.
- ❑ I can clean the refrigerator.
- ❑ I can keep the house clean enough to not be embarrassed when people come.
- ❑ I know where to find manuals and warranties for all appliances.
- ❑ I know where to find phone numbers for repairmen.
- ❑ I know where to find addresses and numbers of friends and relatives.
- ❑ I know where to find records of birthdays, anniversaries, and so forth.
- ❑ I understand my wife's system of bill paying.
- ❑ I am acquainted with her business affairs.
- ❑ I know where to find insurance documents.

Interdependence is perhaps a more descriptive word than independence. You are interdependent, not only in family relationships, but with doctors, bankers, lawyers, friends, and many other people who inhabit your world. It's up to you to choose to be comfortable with yourself and your world as you grow old.

And finally, a section addressed directly to your adult children. You might consider lending them this book, or copying the following pages to send them. If you prefer, you can read the section alone and discuss the ideas that strike you. It can be rewarding to share your reactions with each other. Perhaps you'll find room for further exploration of your changing roles. Perhaps you'll find new grounds for intimacy. Whatever you can share, enjoy the opportunity for contact and connection.

Your Aging Parents — A Section for the Reader's Children

Somehow, when you're young, you don't think the time will ever come when your parents will be old. But here you are with a mother and father who aren't managing very well. Mother is only 70, but she's nearly blind. Dad, at 76, has suddenly become disoriented and unreasonable. He forgets to turn off the stove. Sometimes he forgets to prepare food, and the two of them don't eat for a day. The house is falling into disrepair, and the last time you were there, the roof was leaking. All of a sudden many decisions need to be made. Dad is not mentally competent to make decisions, and mother is so upset by this turn of events that she just wrings her hands and says, "I'm sure it will be all right. Let's don't bother with it now." She is annoyed that you are pressing her to talk about moving out of the house. She is the mother, after all, and you are the child, aren't you? What are you going to do?

Journalist Nancy Friday, in her book, *My Mother, Myself: The Daughter's Search for Identity*, describes the evolution of the mother-daughter relationship over a lifetime. She says that there are phases. The first is clearly the time when mother is mother and child is child. Then come the years of transition, when the two struggle as the child strives for independence and the mother struggles to maintain control. (Do you remember this? It isn't much different for fathers and sons, or sons and mothers, is it?) Ideally, the outcome of this struggle is an adult-adult relationship where the two become friends. Gradually, you find yourselves engaged in a struggle once again as you see the need to protect, nurture, and guide your aging parent. She, or he, resists because that is not at all how she sees her role in life. Hopefully, the outcome will be that you both can accept your changing roles, with mother accepting your care and guidance while you respect her wisdom and wishes. There are six things you can do to ease your mother and father, and yourself, into a workable relationship. I call these the "L Rules": Loving, Listening, License, Learning, Luring, Lauding, and Letting Go.

Loving

Webster's Unabridged Dictionary offers many definitions of the word love, but what matters isn't really semantics or academic definitions. The feelings you have for your parents probably range from devotion to dislike to compassion to an unexplainable and ever-present feeling of responsibility. Aging parents are sometimes a joy, sometimes a burden, often a worry, and always they are a part of you.

Rule of Loving: *Behaving* in a loving way toward another person creates loving feelings.

Another way to think of this rule is, "Acting love creates love." Start by preceding every communication, every decision, and every act with a conscious resolution which you state to yourself — "These are my parents. No matter how difficult it may become, I love them and I will be aware of their needs and their rights." Accompany that with as many hugs and hand squeezes as you can. Human beings of every age thrive on being lovingly touched.

Emily's parents are in good health and still active in their 80s. Recently there have been signs that indicate their need for closer attention. Mom doesn't see as well now, and when she washes dishes they are not always clean. Emily took a bowl from the cupboard and found mold growing in a crack. Once in a while Dad forgets to enter the amount on the checks he has written, so he never knows what the balance is. "It's enough," he'll say.

Emily feels annoyed and disappointed because up until now Dad has always been sharp about money matters. He was the one who taught her to make a budget and manage it. She sees that he needs help but hesitates to override his authority as father. Finally, she was able to approach Dad and say, "Dad, you've helped me so much all the times I had trouble at school or with Bob, and I can't even count the number of times you and Mom have taken care of the kids to give me a break. I really appreciate that. You know, everything I know about money management I learned from you. Would you please let me help you with your checkbook so we can balance the account every month? You know I'm good at it because you taught me." Dad sensed Emily's love and concern and was able to accept her help.

Listening

You can't take care of your parents if you don't hear what they're telling you. Remember when you were 16 and you thought you should be able to take the car whenever you wanted? You probably said, "You don't understand me!" You wanted them to understand your need to be independent. They wanted you to know that their concern for your safety (and the life of the car) didn't mean they didn't trust you.

Sometimes now your parents feel the way you felt at 16 — the need to be listened to and understood. Chapter 3 contains more detailed listening techniques than will be described here, but a brief review may help.

Rule of Listening: I will show my love by listening attentively and helping my parents feel heard and understood.

In brief, these are the steps for good listening:

1. Be able to repeat what your mother or father has said. When you do that, your parent knows you were listening, and you are in a better position to understand.
2. Listen for the *feelings* your parent is conveying. Even though your father may not use words like angry, sad, or lonely, the content of what he is saying can give you a clue. "The days are so long," for instance, probably tells you that he is lonely and sad.
3. Listen for words that indicate a need for help, such as, "I've accumulated so many things during the years — it'll be quite a job to sort it all out."

Test your skill with this example. Choose the response you think is best.

Your mother is having obvious difficulty keeping her balance. You are afraid she will fall when she is alone and perhaps lie injured for hours before she is discovered. When you mention your fear, she says, "I won't fall. I'm always very careful. You don't need to worry about it."

Response:
a: "No matter how careful you are, you still could fall."
b: "That doesn't make sense — of course I worry about you all the time."
c: "I know you're careful, but I can see that your balance is not good."
d: "You don't expect to fall because you're very careful. Sounds like you're confident that you can take care of yourself."

I hope you chose response "d." You have heard what she said, and you have also heard her protecting her independence. This statement lets her know that you understand, and she will be more willing to discuss possible alternatives to her present living situation.

License

In order to drive a car, you have to have a license. If you want to practice medicine or be an electrician, you have to have a license. The license gives you the authority to make decisions and act upon them. Without a license you could make the decision that you need penicillin for your cough, but you would not be able to write the prescription.

By listening to your parents, you give them license to continue to make decisions, and you give yourself license to support their decisions and to help implement them.

Rule of License: I will honor the authority each person has over his or her own rights and responsibilities.

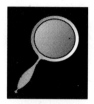 A license implies certain rights and responsibilities. The license also protects your rights and your parents' rights, and ensures that these rights will be exercised responsibly. What are your rights? The exercise on the next page can help you clarify what your rights and responsibilities are, as you see them. The mirror on the left indicates that this is an opportunity for concentrated self-reflection. Look into yourself and into your knowledge of your parents to complete it.

As you think about and complete these lists, why not discuss these issues with your parents? Some of the rights and responsibilities that seem to concern most people are listed below. You will have others, or perhaps the same ones with modifications.

- The right to know that my parents are safe and secure — emotionally, physically, and financially.
- The right to give myself a break from caregiving if I feel myself becoming tense, anxious, or angry.
- The responsibility to be aware of changes in my parents' lives, and to help work out solutions to problems.
- The responsibility to protect my parents from harm of any kind.
- The right to protect their assets insofar as they will allow me.
- The responsibility to provide basic needs in life, such as food, shelter, clothing, and money, when they cannot provide them for themselves.
- The right to provide these things without their consent if they are not competent to understand their own needs.
- Above all else, the right and responsibility to love them, nurture them, and allow them to complete their lives with dignity.

Your parents' rights and responsibilities may sound something like this:

- The right to live where and how they wish, unless their living situation is a threat to their physical well-being.
- The right to expect compassion and understanding as they struggle with the challenges of aging. The right to receive support during times when they cannot be completely independent.
- The right to determine what kind of medical assistance they need and when to refuse it should they choose to do so.
- The right to give their worldly goods to whomever they please.

Rights and Responsibilities

(A Worksheet for Adult Children)

My Rights and Responsibilities

1. I have a right to know that my parents _____

2. I have a right to give myself _____

3. I have a responsibility to _____

4. I have a responsibility to protect _____

5. I have a right to protect _____

6. I have a responsibility to provide _____

7. Above all else, I have a right and a responsibility to _____

8. _____

9. _____

10. _____

11. _____

My Parents Have the Right

1. to live _____

2. to expect _____

3. to receive _____

4. to determine _____

5. to give _____

6. to die _____

7. _____

8. _____

9. _____

My Parents' Responsibilities

1. are primarily to take care of _____

2. to make sure _____

3. to communicate _____

4. _____

5. _____

- The right to die with dignity.
- The responsibility to take care of themselves as long and as well as they can.
- The responsibility to make sure their financial affairs are in order, that they have a living will or trust, and that they have completed unfinished business with other people, if they can.
- The responsibility to communicate to their children and others who may care for them their love and gratitude and their wishes about their final days.

And of course you have to recognize that it isn't just you and your parents, is it? There are other family members, neighbors, friends, clergymen, and a lot of health care professionals who may influence your decisions and who are affected by them. Your license requires that you be aware of these other participants. It also requires you to be responsible for communicating with them. Basically, their right is to be appropriately informed and to be treated with respect. Their responsibility varies with their roles. When you exercise your rights and assume your responsibilities in a way that is respectful of the rights of others, decision making becomes easier.

Learning

The more you know about your parents, the easier it will be to respect and support their decisions. The more you understand your parents, the less painful it will be if you have to make a decision for them. The process of learning about your parents will also provide camaraderie and closeness that you may not have had before. A pleasant side benefit from this experience will be the knowledge you gain about yourself, something valuable for you as you deal with your own aging.

In my naivete as a young woman, I thought it would be nice to have a complete story of my mother's life, so I bought a tape recorder and a pile of tapes and took them to her, expecting that she would spend her evenings talking to the machine. She never recorded one word. She was intimidated by the sound of her own voice. Since then I have talked with others who have had the same experience. I'm doing it differently with my aged aunts. Whenever I talk with them on the phone, I ask a leading question about their youth, or other aspects of life, and then I record the stories they tell. Gradually, I am getting acquainted with them as children, as teens, and as women. Through them I am learning about my mother. I'd like to share with you some of the questions I use.

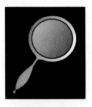 Use the questions on page 188 to help a parent or any loved one reminisce about his or her life experience. The hand mirror to the left reminds you that this is a self-reflection exercise; an opportunity for a closer look into yourself as well as into someone else. Sharing a life story can be moving for both the listener and the narrator. Stay involved by asking questions as you go along.

It's nice to start with the date and other details about his or her birth, and it paves the way for more questions. Please don't wear the older person out with too many questions in one visit.

> **Rule of Learning**: I will show my love through curiosity, and treasure and respect what I learn about my parents.

You may be surprised at the intriguing stories you will hear as you ask these questions. I was enthralled to learn that my husband's aunt was born on a ship during the journey from Denmark. The family settled on Cherry Creek in Denver, and my father-in-law watched the Indian boys at play across the creek.

Once you start talking about memories, all kinds of interesting information will spill forth. For instance, I learned that my aunt was named Walterita because they were expecting a boy to carry on the name of Walter. Understandably, she was not pleased with her name, so she made up one of her own, and she has been know as Carrie all of her life.

When you ask questions about childhood, you can give little prompts now and then to keep things flowing, such as: "What was your house like? Did you have enough money? Tell me about your friends." Other questions will occur to you if you are really listening. It will be hard *not* to get interested in these stories.

When you ask about happy times, it is best to develop the skill of being silent and waiting. It takes a little time for the brain to sift through 70 or 80 years and come up with experiences that were the "best." One friend told me of a time in New York when he just happened to be hanging around outside a large hotel when President Theodore Roosevelt emerged from a limousine. The president shook my friend's hand and left a silver dollar in it.

You may wonder if it's a good idea to let your parents dredge up painful memories about hard times, but it usually is a relief to be able to tell the sad stories to someone who shows interest and who really listens. My mother remembered my grandmother's death during childbirth. Mother was only 13, and at the moment of death she became mother to her younger brothers and sisters. It was a healing experience for her to be able to talk about it.

This process tends to snowball, and you will find yourself asking many questions about details you have not considered before. Maybe you will understand why your parents make decisions in a certain way. Perhaps you will see why some of the things that seem logical and important to you are inconsequential to them, and the other way around. You may even gain insights into your own decision-making process.

Ted

Using Ted for an example, you can see how life events shaped his parents' attitudes about life and death. Ted's parents grew up poor, and they worked hard during their life together to provide decently for the children and make sure they received a college education. Their priorities were not on material things *per se*. Their constant concern was

Learning a Life Story

These questions help you learn more about a person's life experience. Select a few questions at a time, and give your story-teller time to think back. Listen actively, and enjoy what you both discover. Add questions of your own as you listen. There is room to plan additional questions below.

1. Where did your ancestors come from? How did they happen to come to the United States?

2. What do you remember from your childhood about your mother? Grandmother?

3 What do you remember about father? Grandfather?

4. What kind of work did they do?

5. Who named you? Do you know why that name was chosen?

6. What about your brothers and sisters? What were their names? What do you remember about them? Who was older, and who is younger?

7. What was it like when you were a child?

8. Tell me about the happiest times in your life.

9. Were there hard times?

10. Where did you go to school? What was it like?

11. What did you want to be when you grew up?

12. Whom did you admire when you were growing up? Was there someone you wanted to be like?

13. What were birthdays and holidays like? Do you remember any special gifts you gave or received?

14. How did you meet your husband or wife?

15. _____

16. _____

17. _____

18. _____

for the quality of basic needs. They wanted their children to be warm, well fed, curious about everything there was to learn, and to grow up to be compassionate, useful people. They achieved that. There was nothing more they wanted except to watch the grandchildren grow. They were not afraid of dying. Ted's mother grew up accepting death as a stage of life. Ted's father had never been in a hospital, and saw no need ever to go there. They just wanted to live until they died.

Ted struggled within himself, because he valued technology. His idea was that if you got sick, you sought out the best help and applied every possible treatment. The idea was to lick the sickness and beat death. When he fully understood his parents and how they came to hold the values and beliefs they did, he was willing to abide by their wishes.

Luring

In rare instances, parents may not be capable of making decisions. Maybe they lack the intellectual capacity to figure things out. Perhaps there is some organic brain disorder that disables their logical thinking. You will need to be sure that it is not simply a case of being paralyzed by depression and fear, because that can be treated. When it is clearly and irrefutably certain that the problem is organic, such as Alzheimer's or other irreversible brain damage, you may be called upon to make decisions that are not to their liking simply because you must protect them. In this case, you will have to "lure" them.

Luring is not deceitful, nor is it manipulative. Luring is using creative means to teach your parents the good things about the decisions to be made. Most commonly, these decisions involve a change in living arrangements and money management. You may need to obtain a durable power of attorney. Consultation with other family members, health care professionals, and an attorney would be in order before taking this step.

> **Rule of Luring:** When my parents cannot make adequate decisions for themselves, I will present options that appeal to them.

There are three key steps to proper luring:

1. **Assess what is needed**. Do your parents need minimal assistance with daily living tasks, or do they need actual nursing care? Do they have habits that can endanger themselves or others, such as careless smoking, a tendency to leave stove burners on, or wandering away from home? You want to be as objective as possible.

2. **Review your parent's lifestyle**. Have they been gregarious people who love parties and people? Are they quiet folks who like to be left alone with books and

TV? Would they be content in a space that is shared by others? The idea is to consider past evidence to determine likely present preferences.

3. **Make a recommendation**. Based on your assessments, make a recommendation and phrase it in a way most likely to appeal. Explain the benefits in terms of current need and previous preference. Allay fears by acknowledging them and providing reassurance. Find a hook, and make it sound too good to pass up.

Making a careful assessment will help you find the most useful resources. Be sure to consider as many alternatives as possible. If thinking about living options, alternatives might be: living with family members, retirement centers where your parents would be responsible for their own care, retirement centers where meals and housekeeping are provided, assisted living centers, and extended care facilities (which is the euphemism for nursing home). These options were discussed in some detail in the previous chapter.

Any plan you present is going to be met with some resistance. Rather than trying to overcome resistance, work with it. Listen to what your parents are telling you. In order to lure, you have to know their fears and find ways to provide reassurance. Applying pressure to someone who is resistant will only create anger and more resistance. If you meet resistance so strong that you feel blocked, back off and wait. As they feel love, and you demonstrate understanding, they will soften toward your suggestions. Slow and easy is the way to do it. At all times keep this in mind: you are not trying to impose your will upon them — you are trying to solve a problem with them.

May and Her Father

May's father had the habit of smoking in bed, and as he got older he would often drift off to sleep, holding the lighted cigarette. More than once he had awakened to smoldering bedclothes. May noticed the holes in the blankets and in his clothes. She had seen him asleep with hot ash dropping on his clothes. His little house was filthy, and it was a fire hazard. Papers and old magazines were piled everywhere. There were pathways through these piles for getting to the kitchen, the bath, and the bedroom. Many times May had tried to arrange a major cleanup, but Dad would not hear of it. He became extremely angry — red-faced, shouting and cursing. One time he threw an ashtray at May and ordered her out of the house.

May consulted various authorities. The fire department said she could have the house condemned, thus forcing her father to move. Public health officials concurred. Dad's doctor said he could have him hospitalized on a "hold-and-treat" order, and then maybe consider commitment to a state facility, although that would be difficult. May was uncomfortable with all these options. She needed to get Dad somewhere safe. She knew he must have supervision and be assured of good meals and clean linens, but she didn't want him to feel he had been railroaded into what would seem like prison to him. It would be hard to get Dad medically or psychiatrically evaluated because he resisted leaving the house, except for rare occasions when he had an illness that needed treatment. On the other hand, it was frightening to think of him burning the house and himself with it. There was also the danger to other houses nearby. May had no acceptable way to restrict Dad's smoking, either.

After more investigation, May learned that her dad was eligible for acceptance into a special geriatric unit at one of the nursing homes which specialized in Alzheimer's and other organic brain disorders. First, she had to figure out how to pay for it, and then she faced the task of luring her father. Admission to the home was contingent upon medical and psychiatric evaluation. May knew it would be extremely challenging to try to convince Dad to leave his home to live among strangers. How could she make this option attractive?

May talked at length with a social worker at the nursing home, and they devised a plan. Dad loved football and he never missed a televised game. His main complaint in life was that he didn't get the clear reception he would like. The next time May visited Dad, she found him watching Notre Dame destroying Air Force. As usual, he was upset about the fuzzy picture. May watched with him for a while and finally spoke.

May:	You're right, Dad, the reception is terrible. Why, I can hardly tell who the players are.
Dad:	You said it, but there's not a thing we can do about it.
May:	(*asking innocently*) Think you'll ever get cable out here?
Dad:	Not a chance. It'll be the year 3000 before this burg gets modern.
May:	What a shame. You love these games so much. That reminds me — my friend, Sara…you know, she works at Sunshine Towers? Well, I dropped by to see her the other day, and she was watching the C.U.–Nebraska game. It was like being right there, the picture was so clear. I could just about smell the popcorn.
Dad:	(*looking at May disbelievingly*) She was watching on the job?
May:	Oh yes. Her office is right beside the family room, so she steps out now and then to see what's going on.
Dad:	Family room? I thought Sunshine Towers was a rest home.
May:	Oh no, Dad, it's just an apartment building where only people over 60 can live. It's next door to the rest home.
Dad:	I don't get it.
May:	Well, each person has his own apartment, but there is also a great big family room that everyone can use. It's nice because they have a fireplace, and a huge TV — bigger than anyone could afford to have in their own living room — and you can play cards or read.
Dad:	(*interested*) I'll bet that costs an arm and a leg.

The door was open for luring Dad out of his filthy house and into a structured living situation in which he could not only have privacy and freedom, but also supervision. Paying attention to what Dad enjoyed most in life was the key.

Lauding

Most people thrive on praise and recognition. Children blossom when praised and encouraged, but shrivel when criticized. Those who are older also thrive on praise, but when belittled or criticized tend to become obstinate. Your parents are probably no exception. If you are supportive of their decisions, whether those decisions appeal to you or not, they are more likely to make decisions that are agreeable to both of you.

> **Rule for Lauding:** I will point out things that are pleasing and keep silent about things I don't like in my parents, unless something interferes with my rights and responsibilities.

This rule for lauding is the respectful way to treat anyone, and your parents deserve it most of all. It doesn't mean keeping silent when your toes are stepped on, or when you believe a certain behavior might lead to danger. But it does mean focusing on the positive, and refraining from criticism whenever you can. When you must criticize, remember to use "I" statements. You are pointing out a problem to *you*, not a problem in your parent. If you think the problem is a fundamental one in your parent, bite your tongue. Such criticism won't bring change.

Sara, the social worker, invited May and her dad to have lunch with her at Sunshine Towers. Dad was reluctant at first, but included in the invitation was an opportunity to spend the afternoon watching a game. May said to her dad, "I'm happy to be going to lunch with *my Dad*. I admire your adventurous spirit." Dad was given an opportunity to see how he would benefit by moving into a protected environment, and he decided he liked the idea well enough that he would go through the interviews and examinations. At no time did May coerce or threaten. The final decision was Dad's. He never knew of the possibility of having his house condemned or the threat of hospitalization. May congratulated him on each decision and expressed her pleasure at his happiness. She carefully avoided criticism or derogatory remarks about the way he had been living.

Letting Go

And finally, there comes a day when you have done the best you could, and no matter what the consequences are, you have to live with either the decisions your parents made or the decisions you were forced to make for them. This is very hard. You want your parents to have a nice life, and sometimes it doesn't work out.

> **Rule of Letting Go**: I can only do so much for other people. Once I have done my best to help, I must let them lead their own lives.

At the age of 85, my husband's aunt developed a large ulcer on her leg. It was thought to be the result of poor circulation, and she refused medical treatment. The ulcer got worse. She was in terrible pain, and she was ill. Finally, we felt we had to override her wishes and put her into a hospital. Many tests were done, and it was determined that there was no circulation at all to that leg. She had gangrene and would die if the leg were not amputated. She hated the hospital, and she was angry with me for taking her there. "Why did you have to take over?" she asked me. When the doctor approached her with the idea of amputation, she was adamant. "No!" she said firmly. The doctor explained that she could probably get well without the bad leg. He told her she would die if she kept the leg. "No amputation," she said, "and take this thing out of my nose." Tanta had not been able to eat because she was too sick, and so a feeding tube had been put in. There were conferences: the doctors, psychiatrist, my husband, and myself...with and without Tanta. We agreed that she was competent to make the decision, so we had to abide by it. Her primary doctor went back to the bedside. "Miss Birkedahl," he said, "do you understand what will happen if we don't take your leg off?"

"Yes," she said, looking him straight in the eye. "I don't want my leg cut off. Just let me go home to mother." (Mother had been dead some 20 years.)

"Do you want the tube taken out of your nose?" he asked.

Tanta took his hand and said, with pleading in her voice, "Oh yes, please!"

I sat with Tanta the night she died and talked about Christmases we had when the children were small. I told her that I knew she was leaving us, and that it was OK. I told her how much we loved her. She squeezed my hand, and I knew I was forgiven.

I'm still not certain that anything we did was right, but I don't know that it was wrong, either. I just know that there comes a time when you have to decide to let go.

A resource which may be helpful to you is Children of Aging Parents (CAPS). This organization serves as a national resource clearing house for caregivers. They offer a national network of support groups, workshops, and seminars. CAPS also offers advice and informational leaflets. For more information, send $1 with a self-addressed, stamped envelope to CAPS, 2761 Trenton Road, Levittown, PA 19056.

This chapter suggested various ways of adjusting and strengthening your family's ties. At times this means setting limits, especially when you continue to spend a great deal of time together. But usually this means reaching out — continuing to learn about, understand, and respect each member of your family network. The family is a miniature society; it is the buffer between the larger society and you. In the next chapter, you will focus on ways to become more involved in the larger society. But a strong family provides you with both a springboard and a safety net as you reach further out. Strong doesn't mean "ideal"; it just means working to change as needed, and bound by love.

References

Erikson, E., J.M. Erikson, and H.Q. Kivnick. (1986) *Vital Involvement in Old Age.* New York and London: W.W. Norton and Co.

Fontana, A. (1977) *The Last Frontier: The Social Meaning of Growing Old.* Beverly Hills, CA, and London: Sage Publications.

Friday, N. (1977) My Mother, Myself: The Daughter's Search for Identity. New York: Delacorte Press.

Fromme, A. (1984) *60+ Planning It, Living It, Loving It.* New York: Farrar, Strauss and Giroux.

Trieschmann, R.B. (1987) *Aging With a Disability.* New York: Demos Publications.

Weiner, M., J. Teresi, and C. Streich (1983) *Old People Are a Burden, But Not My Parents.* Englewood Cliffs, N J: Prentice-Hall, Inc.

9

Getting Involved

So far you have been looking at yourself in the rather narrow sense of you as a person, your inner systems, and your family. There is a tendency for a lot of people to keep their lives confined to this narrow perspective. I was talking to a 75-year-old man the other day and he said, "I used to drive all over the United States, now I can't drive much at all. I can't ride my bike or walk very far, I feel like I'm in a cage, confined to my own back yard."

This chapter is about broadening your interests and expanding your outlook. You're going to open the door of the cage and examine the world. There are people who have an adventuresome spirit and the resources to physically go out and explore the world. There are others who are restricted by disability or low income who can't fly to Africa or take a boat to Greece. No matter, you are still a part of the world and the universe. You have a special place in it and a contribution to make. Your life will be greatly enriched from reaching out, from learning, and from doing.

Reaching Out

In Chapter 1, you made an assessment of your inner systems. Chapter 2 suggested you begin to look outward, to the network of family and friends that anchor you in the world. It's now time to examine issues and events locally, nationally, and globally. These systems are part of your larger support network; together, all create a universal living system. Refer to the Complete Living Systems Inventory in Chapter 2 as you work through this chapter; you'll have a chance to create a larger, more thorough inventory later. It can be exciting to broaden your focus. In the process of getting to know the larger world around you, you'll have ample opportunity to become involved.

If you have been involved in solving problems at some level, you know the rewards it presents. Why not look at other levels and see what steps you might take to improve things there? If you haven't gotten involved yet, now's the time to start.

Service Beyond the Family

You are a citizen, and you have a responsibility that doesn't end with old age. It ends only with death. Unless you are at this moment confined to your bed, totally paralyzed, and drawing your last breath, there is something you can do. If you can think, you can do.

It's simple, but it's not easy. A basic fact of life is that at every age there is a drive to do, a need to serve. Some people cling to their children, failing to let go of the parental role, using the children as their only vehicle for service. No one would question the idea that you never stop serving your family, one way or another. Of course family always needs you in some capacity, as you need them. But this doesn't mean creating a situation that encourages adult children to remain dependent. When that happens, you automatically restrict yourself to a cage of your own making. Worse than that, you restrict your children and stifle their growth.

You can help your adult children to maintain independence by capitalizing on assets — theirs and yours. There are two ways to do that. One is to constantly reinforce your children's assets, perhaps by saying, "I admire your strength and your artistic ability; I think you can use that in many different occupations." The second approach is more direct: "Because I see that you have strength and ability, I cannot encourage you to waste it. I want you to be out in the world building a life for yourself, for that is where you will find happiness."

It is not fair to limit your giving to the family when they are struggling to become independent. Give the children the opportunity to struggle and survive on their own. Your talents and your need to serve can now be extended to the world around you.

The Wealth of Age

However you can reach out, your life will be brighter for it. Your community needs your wisdom and experience. It needs leaders. The richest storehouse for finding people with leadership skills is the growing population of older people: people like you. If you think that you don't have leadership skills, you haven't taken a good look at your life.

You've raised a family, either with a spouse or alone. You've made plans and carried them out. You know how to manage money. There have been emergencies of various sorts that you learned how to handle. You have a lifetime of learning in your brain — book learning, classroom learning, job learning, and the wonderful learning that comes from experience. You are knowledgeable and wise.

What you must do is refuse to be relegated to the role of "elderly" as it is defined by society. There is a much truer and more positive definition of elderly. An *elder* is a person who has authority, someone who is superior in rank and validity. An elder has wisdom and dignity. How do you find the way to use your elder abilities? Start with something you are interested in that will use a specific skill you already have, or one that will allow you to learn a new skill.

Naomi

Naomi has rheumatoid arthritis. Her hands are badly twisted, and she can barely walk. In spite of the crippling effects of the disease on her hands, Naomi can knit. To look at her hands you would never think it was possible. One project she was particularly interested in was providing winter clothing for homeless families. She was especially concerned about the children, who would be going to school feeling unhappy and out of place. She discussed a plan with her husband, Rex.

Naomi:	Those kids need to look nice.
Rex:	Sure they do, but I don't see what we can do about it. We barely make it each month as it is. The heat bill's been so high that I'm not even sure we can pay that.
Naomi:	I know, but look, Rex [*showing him a sack of leftover yarn*]. This is all from sweaters I used to make for our boys. I could make warm caps, brightly colored caps for the children.

The days passed quickly as Naomi met her goal of one cap each week. By December she had 10 caps of varied colors and designs, some with pompoms, some with stocking tails.

Naomi:	OK, Rex, I'm ready to go.
Rex:	Go where?
Naomi:	Down to the place where they're collecting clothes for the homeless.
Rex:	I can run those down for you.
Naomi:	No sir, I'm looking forward to taking them in myself.

The women at the distribution center were pleased to have the caps. They commented on the excellent workmanship and the combinations of colors. One woman said, "Ten children are going to go to school warm and happy." Another looking at Naomi's work commented, "No one else will have a cap as fine as this." And a third woman asked Naomi, "Would you like to do another project?"

Naomi found that her skills were needed, and that being disabled didn't mean she couldn't help others.

Making a Plan

As you work through this chapter you are likely to come across events you'd like to support or organizations that need help. Having a plan will facilitate your efforts. You need to know, realistically, what you are able to do. You need to recognize what types of things you'd like to do, and ways to go about it. Considering the questions below can help you begin.

1. What resources do I have that will enable me to participate in the world around me? (Consider money, physical strength, special skills such as typing, bookkeeping, marketing, and so forth. Perhaps you have equipment you could loan or donate. Check your list of personal assets from Chapter 2 for more ideas about how to participate.) _____

_____

_____

_____

2. What skills or interests have proved to be rewarding throughout my life?_____

_____

_____

_____

3. What new skills or interests might I develop now that I never had a chance to before? _____

_____

_____

4. What are my limitations? (physical, financial, time, energy) _____

_____

_____

_____

5. With this ratio of resources to limitations, where can I realistically begin to cultivate my interests? (For ideas, see the list below.) _____

_____

_____

_____

6. Who, besides me, might benefit? _____

_____

_____

_____

You can develop motivation and enthusiasm by using a visualization to remember a time when you felt rewarded by the successful use of one or more of your skills. As you do this, you will see how your skills can be newly applied to a volunteer project now. Last night I attended a dinner which was given by the symphony board to show appreciation for the musicians in the orchestra. A woman there told me she became involved with symphony fund raising because she remembered how much fun it was in high school to sell calendars so the choir could take a trip to Disneyland.

One way to match the above to reality is to consider the list included below, and to open your phone book. From the list, select two or three agencies that sound interesting. Find the local equivalent in the phone book, call and see if they need volunteers, and then go there and ask how they would plan to use you. Don't commit yourself until you've looked things over. Assess whether those in charge are people you'd like to work with every week. See if the work is something you can handle, physically and emotionally.

It may be that you will be more interested in finding a place that can help you develop a skill before you think of volunteering. Many places that value volunteers offer free training, either through a formal program or a more informal appprenticeship. Feel free to ask about training when you approach an organization as a volunteer.

Organizations Seeking Volunteers

Alcoholics Anonymous	Hospitals
Arthritis Foundation	Libraries
Cancer Society	Mental Health Centers
Centers for Deaf and Blind	Nursing Homes
Community Symphony Orchestras	Older American Centers
Crisis Helplines	Planned Parenthood Center
Foster Grandparents	Professional Symphony Orchestras
Gray Gourmet	RSVP (Retired Senior
Hospices	Volunteer Program)

There are many more organizations and causes that could use your help. The Resources section at the end of this book include some volunteer organizations that will help guide your search. In the process of searching, you may come across some unique group that will be just what you want.

Keeping a Journal

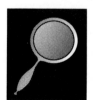 As you begin to experiment with new uses for your skills, it's a good idea to keep a journal of your experiences. Journal writing is the best way I know to realize emotional growth from daily life. As you write, your experiences become knowledge, and after a while they become wisdom. It's like planting seeds. At first it's just words on paper, but after a period of time you develop insights. These new thoughts grow, like the lovely plants that spring from the seeds. Things to include in your journal, if you've never kept one before, might be the day's activities and your feelings about them, goals you've been thinking about, conversations that were meaningful, disappointments you experienced that day, and memories that were triggered by the day's events.

Here are some excerpts from Cathy's journal. Cathy had loved to paint as a little girl but it had been decades since she held a brush. Her journal reflects the anxiety she felt when she decided to take the plunge and develop her long-dormant artistic skills.

Cathy's Journal

Sept. 3

Today was my first art class. I was so eager for it to begin, and then on the way there I began to fear that my efforts would be laughable. Would the others think I was a foolish old woman for being there? What a relief to find that the other six people in my class had no drawing experience. We all laughed at our first attempts, and it was fun. The teacher is a nice man who really is an artist, but he seemed to enjoy our laughter, too. Now I have *homework*.

Sept. 5

Today I drew an apple that actually looked like an apple. It's kind of flat, one dimensional, but you can tell it's an apple. It's fun, it's like letting something out of the inside of me that's been bottled up for a long, long time.

Oct. 14

They want volunteers at the art center. I think I'd like to do that, but I have my usual fear of looking foolish. I'm noticing that this has been a pattern in my life. I've been afraid of doing things for fear of being laughed at, and boy, I've missed out on a lot.

Oct. 16

I signed up to be a volunteer. They said they'd love to have me because I love art. Isn't that amazing? They didn't care that I don't have a background in art, they just care that I love it. I do love it.

Oct. 25

Today they asked me to go to an elementary school and explain about the children's art contest. Of course my first thought was will I look foolish, but it only lasted a flash. My next thought was gee, how neat. I'm getting over those silly fears. I'm doing better with my drawing, too. The things I draw look round instead of flat. I like my drawings; they are me. That's the main thing — I'm me and I don't need to try to be what some person in my imagination thinks I should be. Actually, I don't think anyone is expecting me to be anything. Hooray, what freedom!

Cathy's personal growth is apparent. She is moving out of her cloistered, timid lifestyle. She's developing latent talents and learning about herself in the process. That's what community service usually does for people, but sometimes they don't gain the insights if they're not writing things down.

The Larger Systems

Widening your circle to service at a state, national, or world level may seem intimidating. It's probably unrealistic to aspire to be governor or president of the United States, but there are many avenues for service. You never know what might happen once you get involved.

I have a friend whose daughter has epilepsy. When the child was young, Denise became involved in the local chapter of the epilepsy association because she needed help for herself. She simply couldn't handle having this terrible thing happen to her little girl. Less was known 40 years ago, and the social stigma was stronger. Denise put a lot of energy into the organization because she saw that others suffered the same pain she was experiencing. Over time, Denise became president of the local group, then president of the state group, and finally, after her husband died, she became regional director — a paid position which necessitated a move to a larger city. When Denise started out, she had no thought of taking on a leadership role, she simply needed help in a situation that was overwhelming.

That's not necessarily what will happen to you when you get involved as a volunteer on the local level. Something similar could happen, and you would be the most surprised person of all if it did. The point is, however, that community service opens doors. You can walk through them or not, as you please.

Community

What things do you like about your community? How are the streets? Are there sidewalks wide enough for walking? Is it a safe place for an older person to live? Are there stores and doctors and banks nearby? These are important considerations. You need to think about how long you'll be driving and how costly and available public transportation is. On whom do you depend in emergencies? Communities also have personalities, just like people. Is your community attractive or is it so dingy that it gets you down? Are people in your area friendly or do they keep to themselves, remaining anonymous?

Answering all of these questions will help you form a profile of your community. Other things to explore would be services for seniors, such as Gray Gourmet and Older American Centers. These centers go by many names but they're not hard to find. Usually, both Gray Gourmet and the Older American Centers have a list of menus and activities in the calendar section of your newspaper. You can also look up AARP (American Association of Retired Persons) in the phone book. They can give you more information about special services.

After you have a comprehensive picture of your community, you will be able to make decisions about whether to move or stay. If you decide to stay, you can then go through the process of finding ways to get involved in making your community better. That brings you full circle...back to volunteer work.

If you decide there is nothing you can do to make your community a good place to live, then you have the option of moving. In that case, you would go through the same process described above for each community you are considering. You could even take these questions and concerns and put them into the form of a questionnaire that you could carry around with you. Perhaps a checklist including such questions as: Is the bank easy to get to? __Yes __No. This is a technique that will be useful for many decisions you will need to make which have not been covered in this book. You may also want to draw up balance sheets, or inventories, as you did for the living systems discussed in Chapters 1 and 2. The next section will show you how to set them up for larger living systems. Mary Ann has had some experiences that may interest you.

Mary Ann

Mary Ann lives in a neighborhood of 30-year-old homes, mostly occupied by middle-aged people, with a scattering of young families and a couple of older folks like herself. By and large the people are friendly but never seem to get very well-acquainted. Mostly they visit when they're out in their yards, but they don't know much about each other. It's a good neighborhood in many ways. The yards are kept up pretty well. There's a bank three blocks away. The largest hospital is nearby. Two grocery stores grace the area, so it has many assets.

There are a few liabilities. This community contains a large high school. It seems that every student, no matter how near or far away he or she lives, drives to school. The parking lot isn't big enough, so the students park on the nearby residential streets. Even so, the assets outweigh the liabilities.

Mary Ann doesn't know the names of everyone on the block, and has only been in her neighbors' homes briefly when collecting for the cancer society. One day she looked out and saw a white-haired woman walking down the middle of the street. She was rather unkempt, and seemed to be lost. "Can this be a bag person who has wandered up from the other side of town," Mary Ann wondered? No, she wasn't carrying anything. Mary Ann went out and asked if she could help. The woman indicated that she wanted to go over to the high school. This was puzzling. Then the woman pointed to a house across the street and said that was where she wanted to go. By this time, Mary Ann knew that the woman did not know where she was or what she wanted to do. All she knew for sure was her name, Gracie.

Mary Ann escorted Gracie to her car and headed for the local hospital. She didn't know what to expect there, but was greeted by a nurse who listened to the story.

The nurse was miraculously able to obtain Gracie's last name. The clerk went back over hospital records and found a recent admission. He was able to produce the name of Gracie's sister, with whom she lived, and her address. Imagine Mary Ann's chagrin when she learned that Gracie lived two doors down the street from her own home.

"To think that I never even knew there was another person living in that house," she said. "That's a liability for me, personally, as well as for the neighborhood, and certainly for Gracie."

The sister later told Mary Ann that she had to keep Gracie in the house with the doors locked. Gracie had Alzheimer's disease and was disposed to walk out and wander, with no regard for cars, traffic lights, or even whether she was appropriately dressed. Shortly after this incident, the sister started taking Gracie to an adult daycare program three mornings a week.

"Well, that's an asset," Mary Ann said, "to have a place in our community for Gracie to go for socialization."

Mary Ann made a decision to visit Gracie once a week. Over time, Gracie remembered her and looked forward to her coming. This led Mary Ann to wonder if there were other shut-ins who might enjoy a friendly visit, so she contacted the home health department at the hospital and signed up as a volunteer.

Mary Ann recorded her thoughts on the inventory that follows.

Living Systems Inventory

Community

Mary Ann

Assets	Liabilities	Resources
Attractive houses and yards. Friendly people. Bank close by. Hospital near. Grocery store near.	People stay inside; not much interaction between neighbors. I don't even know all the neighbors. High school brings noise, traffic.	Hospital with helpful staff, good referral capabilities. Adult daycare center (for Gracie).

What I Can Do

Make an effort to meet more neighbors. (Maybe collect for other charities?)
Volunteer at hospital.
Reach out to other elders in need of outside care and supervision. (This can be point of contact with other neighbors.)

You'll notice that the last section, "What I Can Do," is space to brainstorm further on volunteer opportunies. As you look around at *your* community, you will probably find unique assets, unique liabilities, and strong resources. You may find that some assets are also liabilities (just like with people). Keep track of your thoughts on the inventory that follows. Remember to think about possible roles for yourself in everything you write.

State

In one sense, a state is a larger community, but there are dramatic differences. There are more legislative activities, more rules and regulations, and more taxes than you have at the local level. How much do you know about your state government? Is it effective?

Living Systems Inventory

Community

Assets	Liabilities	Resources

What I Can Do

Is there concern for the needs of your age group? What do you like about your state? What things do you wish were different?

First, think about all the things you already know about your state. You can begin to fill in assets and liabilities on the state inventory. What products or qualities is your state famous for, and how do you feel about them? Are there things you wish you could find in your state but you can't? You may want to become better acquainted with your state by reading about its history and making trips to historically interesting sites. Libraries and museums are great stores of information. I ought to warn you, though, that this sort of thing is fascinating and quite addictive. You might end up writing a book!

Maybe there are things about your state that you would change if you could. The state is the first larger system where laws made far from your home can impact you directly. Of course, you can still play an active role in that law-making process.

Have you ever attended a legislative session? For that matter, have you ever attended city council or town meetings? These things may be worth your while — especially if issues of concern to you are under discussion. You might even want to *introduce* issue if you feel they are not receiving enough attention. Your voice counts, but it's up to you to make sure it's heard

Making Yourself Heard

The essential act of living in a democracy is voting. In each election, you are given the right to select your own representatives to speak on your behalf. That's why understanding the issues and the candidates' positions is so important. If you don't decide who or what is best for you, your state, or your nation, someone else will.

+---

Living Systems Inventory

State

Assets	Liabilities	Resources

What I Can Do

Voting is a first step, but you can do more. Attending legislative sessions or visiting senators is an option for those who can do so. If you can't travel, but still care what goes on in your behalf, the single most important thing you can do is to write letters to those who make the laws. As few as 100 letters received by any member of State or Federal Congress is enough to make a lawmaker take notice. He, or she, might be strongly enough impressed to change his vote. The way to write the letter is this:

1. State that you have learned of a proposal being considered. Give the name and number of the bill if you can.
2. State that you support the proposal.
3. Explain briefly why you support it.
4. Ask for the senator's or representative's vote.
5. Express appreciation for their service.
6. Address your letter to The Honorable _____, Senate Office Building, your state capitol.

Follow the same procedure at the national level, addressing it in the same way to Washington, D.C. 20510.

Jim

While on a business trip to the state capital, Jim decided to attend a legislative session. He was still struggling to work through his grief over his wife's death and thought this might help him think about something else. On that particular day, the legislature was discussing water. Some parts of the state have plenty of water, other areas are parched. As Jim listened to the discussion, he was surprised to learn that there are many more issues at stake than just distributing water. He decided to learn more about it.

He started with the public library, and that led him to the university, and from there to legal archives. Finally, he wound up in a senator's office to ask questions. Jim never in the world expected to do such a thing. The result of the interview was that Jim had a broader view of his state, more than just water rights. He recognized himself as an important part of the system. He began to write letters to national environmental concerns — and solicited friends to do likewise. He is no longer a passive bystander talking about what "they" have done. "They" has become "me." Jim is doing all he can to improve his current world — and leave a better one for those who came after him.

Nation

All the issues at the state level are amplified at the national level. Federal laws affect you, obviously. Government agencies have policies which may have special meaning for you. Some, you may not even be aware of. Others have been an ongoing concern.

The assets and liabilities are larger, more complex, and the resources may be more tedious to access. You can begin by listing them as you know them at this time in your life. What things *have* you used or been proud of or been irritated by? What does America mean to you?

When you consider your nation, larger issues come into play then at other levels. Most people have deep feelings about their nation. Were you born in the United States, or did you come here from another country? If you came from another place, what have you gained by coming to the United States? What have you lost? Whether you were born here or came from somewhere else, you have been through a lot and have many experiences to tell. Use the following self-reflection exercise for deepening your perception of the nation. The questions are open-ended, for you to interpret as you like.

1. In general, I believe the United States is_____
    _____
    _____

2. There are certain aspects of government that concern me, especially ___
    _____

_____

3. The president _____
    _____

    _____

4. When I was young, things were different. I remember _____
    _____

    _____

5. The biggest changes I've seen are _____
    _____

Living Systems Inventory

Nation

Assets	Liabilities	Resources

What I Can Do

6. What I would like to see changed now is _____
_____
_____

7. The ways in which I might create change are _____
_____
_____

Being informed is the first step to action. There are many ways to have an effect, such as being an informed voter, working with the League of Women Voters, or for your favorite political candidate. If you drive, you could provide transportation for those who have difficulty getting to the polls. And writing letters is still a potent instrument for change. List the assets and liabilities of your country just as you did for yourself, family, community, and state. Consider emotional and sentimental issues as well. Some of the decisions you will soon be facing will require you to understand government policies. You can use governmental resources to your advantage if you understand them.

World

There are people who subscribe to an isolationist policy for the United States. It's a tempting thought, in a way. Why get involved with other countries and their troubles? But it isn't that simple. In my opinion, isolationism won't work. The United States is a part of the world. You are a part of the world, just as your left lung is a part of you. You have lived through more than one war. You may have lost a child in a war, or a husband, or a wife. Your grandchildren are facing the threat of war. War and other experiences from the past affect you today. So many things go into your understanding of the planet around you. This discussion touches on a few different ways you might think about and experience the world. International politics; personal memories; environmental concerns; travel; TV news stories — see which of these sections capture your way of connecting with the world. That perspective will help you when you begin to fill out your Living Systems Inventory, *World*.

War Memories

Walt is someone I know well, having lived with him for over 40 years. Walt understands things through experience and analogy. In World War II, he was a glider pilot who landed behind enemy lines in the major invasion into Normandy, Holland, and Germany. His ability to survive depended upon knowledge of the terrain, skill in landing the glider safely, knowing how to return to his unit without getting shot or captured, and a lot of luck. And that is the way Walt approaches life today at age 71. He believes in being prepared, increasing his skills, and recognizing the unpredictability of circumstances that are not under his control. Walt just has an "Oh well, here goes nothing," attitude. He might not have lived in quite this way if he had not had the war experience. War colors his understanding of the world. There are many liabilities in war. There can be assets, too. The asset for Walt was the development of an attitude about life that enables him to make adjustments to his constantly changing internal and external environment. It also makes him a pleasant and durable companion. He has written of his experiences in an unpublished book called "G is for Guts." He wrote it for his grandchildren.

Frieda, too, was touched by war: she grew up in Berlin. Although her war experience isn't constantly on her mind, it does affect her behavior today. Frieda remembers World War II vividly. She recalls how she was trained to fall to the ground and lie flat at the first sound of a whistle or siren. Later, after she came to the United States, she became professor of psychology at a large university. In 1976, she was invited to give a workshop in a small town in the mountains of Colorado. In this town, it had long been the custom to blow a loud whistle at noon. In the early days, it was for the purpose of telling miners to take a lunch break. If it blew at any other time, it meant there had been an accident in the mine. The mines are closed now, but they still blow the noon whistle. It's part of the local color. The morning session of Frieda's workshop adjourned at 11:30. She was standing with some students discussing where to go for lunch when suddenly the whistle sounded and Frieda found herself flat on the sidewalk. It was an automatic response, programmed in during those days of terror. This event occurred 40 years after the war was over. Can you think how some of the things you do, or attitudes you have, came from past events?

Current Events

Events in remote places may be an asset or liability to you, personally. With today's communication network, images of world events come directly into your living room.

Documentaries capture international tales of grief; news flashes confront you with distant but immediate triumphs and horrors. It's hard not to react personally. There are many thousands of starving children in the world, whose images haunt me at night. I can't think of an asset weighty enough to counterbalance this liability. Are there world news images that have struck you deeply?

When you think about those situations, you may want to look for ways to help. By doing research you might find that there are tasks needing doing which would facilitate the adoption of children in the world who are neglected. Money is always welcome, but there is volunteer work that you could do. Agencies exist specifically to match interested people with needy causes. See what your local yellow pages list under International Aid or Social Services.

Eleanor Roosevelt once said, "I could not at any age be content to take my place in a corner by the fireside and simply look on. Life was meant to be lived. One must never, for whatever reason, turn one's back on life." This much-traveled lady was well-informed about world affairs. Oh sure, you say, she was a president's wife, she had money and opportunities. The point is, it would not have mattered who Eleanor Roosevelt was married to, she would have been interested in everything that was going on in the world whatever her station in life. It seems to me that each of us is one part of a large whole.

Has your experience and perspective given you insight that could be shared with others? Children, teenagers, and college students need to hear their elders talk about their experiences. Politicians must know what your ideas are — without them they cannot serve you well. Letters to the editor are good for voicing opinions, and those letters are read by people who often don't bother with the news articles.

Can You Save the Planet?

More and more people are becoming aware of the planet as a precariously balanced ecological miracle. One person does not have much control over how much carbon monoxide is in the air, or whether the ozone will be depleted. One hundred thousand people making small efforts have a great deal of control over both of those things. When you develop awareness of the small acts that can make a difference, then you are in control of what happens to the earth.

One of my favorite books on this subject is Jeffrey Hollender's *How to Make the World a Better Place*. Hollender says, "The shape of the future is in our hands. It is our responsibility, for it can be no one else's." This statement is particularly applicable to the elders in our society. It is the elders who teach by their example how to take care of this world. The elders are the ones who have time and experience to do the things that will make a difference.

Have you ever witnessed a destructive act and thought to yourself, "I should report that, but others have seen it, someone else has already done it"? The trouble with that kind of thinking is that everyone else may be thinking the way you are. It's really up to us, you and me, to be the guardians and protectors of the environment.

The first and most obvious thing to do is to look at your own habits. Do you leave the water running while brushing your teeth or shaving? If you turn the faucet on only when actually using the water, you will save thousands of gallons of water every year. Do you turn off the lights when you leave a room? That simple act alone will have significant impact on energy resources.

Do you get the car out to drive three blocks to the grocery? Could you walk if you're only getting a few things? And while you're there, how about buying recycled tissues and paper towels?

Think of all the foods that come in styrofoam packages. You could look for things that are packaged in better materials, such as paper. Do you take your own bags to the grocery, or are you accumulating a huge number of paper bags by getting new ones each time?

Small things, yes, but important acts of conservation. You are probably doing all of these things and more even now. Look beyond your present pattern of conservation, try to find more ways to become involved. There are thousands of such acts, but this book is not the place to list them all. My goal is to encourage you to be aware of how what you do affects your world.

Living Systems Inventory

World

Assets	Liabilities	Resources
What I Can Do		

Getting Ready

The natural world is not a quiet place. Natural disasters take us by surprise. Tornadoes, hurricanes, hail, and floods cannot always be predicted with accuracy. There are two things you can do as a citizen of this unpredictable system to be prepared for disaster. First, you can have your own affairs in order, and second, you can become involved in helping others.

An example of having your own household in order would be the common event of a broken water main. You know what happens when the doorbell rings and it turns out to be a workman telling you that the water will be shut off for several hours. You can avoid the frantic filling of pans and buckets if you store 15 or 20 bottles of water for when the emergency arises.

It's also a good idea to have food storage. Buy extras of the things you like to eat, date them, and store them. It's not good to have canned foods sitting on a shelf for years and years, so use your food storage and replenish it often, placing the newly purchased items behind existing ones. Many people store enough food for a year, which can be a lifesaver if your social security checks stop coming or your town is wiped out by a tornado. I encourage you to at least store enough food, toilet tissue, and water for 72 hours. That is about how long it takes for emergency relief efforts to become effective. More information is available by contacting some of the organizations in the Resources section at the end of the book.

In the summer of 1990, the town of Limon, Colorado, was destroyed by a tornado. The bank became a pile of rubble, stores were literally blown off the foundations and scattered to the four winds. Houses were completely destroyed. They didn't expect it, they weren't prepared for it, and it was a disaster of the first order. For an older person caught in that kind of destruction it can be a matter of life and death. Being homeless, without food and necessary medications, is a situation not tolerated well by elders.

Thousands of people donated money, food, furniture, and clothing to the people of Limon. Materials for rebuilding were made available. If you are aware of disasters occurring locally or in far places, you can find ways to help. You just have to look for them.

More immediately you can organize a community effort of preparedness. Get together with your neighbors and make a plan for disaster. How can community resources be called into play? Who will be responsible for notifying authorities? Who has readily available transportation to help in evacuation? As you discuss the possibilities, you will find many more questions arising. Get your plan on paper and help people commit to certain tasks.

Venturing Out

The world has become a very accessible place. Some people get to know the world around them by actually visiting and exploring its every corner. If you like to travel and have the means, then by all means do so. I hope you're not putting off a dream trip until some "better" day. The better day may not come. An old friend of our family dreamed of a trip to Europe. He and his wife spent quite a lot of time looking at timetables and brochures, planning their trip. Each year he said, "If we wait until next year, we'll have more money, and then we can do the trip in style." Each year his wife grew more frail. This went on for about 15 years. Then his wife died. He said to us, "If there's someplace you really want to go, do it now. Otherwise you may not get the chance. You may not have the luxuries you would have if you waited until you had more money, but at least you'll realize your dream." He didn't want to go to Europe without his wife, and so he just went on working until he, too, succumbed to a final illness.

Major trips such as my friend described are not always possible, or even desirable. There are other ways to expand your mind and stimulate your imagination. Reading about other countries is almost as exciting as being there. I've always had a yen to go to Georgia, but it's never worked out, so I wrote to the Chamber of Commerce in several cities and received colorful booklets about everything interesting in Georgia.

Small trips, closer to home, have as much value and considerably more comfort than long-distance trips. There are also economy trips for elders through the American Association of Retired Persons (AARP). Bus tours with a group are fun, and some people who have motor homes or campers enjoy traveling along with a group. Elder Hostel sponsors trips, and they also provide educational opportunities at colleges, giving you the pleasure of a trip as well as a chance to learn. (See the list of Resources at the end of the book for information on contacting these agencies.)

I know a number of people who have specialized training in music, art, geology, or history, who have volunteered to be tour guides. That way you get the trip paid for. It would be fun to do the research in preparation for such a job. You can investigate that by talking to travel agency personnel or to the public relations department at your local college or university.

If you do decide to travel, here are some hints that make a trip more fun:

1. Plan to travel only as far as you can comfortably handle each day.
Pushing to make a certain number of miles can jeopardize your health.

2. Make your preparations well in advance.
Don't leave shopping and packing and hair-cutting until the last week. Get everything ready and then spend the last week resting, watering plants, telling your neighbor you'll be gone. Most important...go to bed early for a week!

3. Take only the absolute necessities.
Don't buy a lot of new clothes. Leave your best dresses and shirts at home. Take the old ones. When they get dirty, discard them. If you need more clothes, buy them on the trip instead of before. Sounds wasteful, but it'll make your trip a lot easier.

4. Take enough doses of medicine for the number of days you'll be gone plus for one day extra.
Ask your doctor for prescriptions, including eyeglass prescriptions, and a letter about any medical problem you have that could get you into trouble. If you have to go to a doctor or clinic, request that the doctor call your own doctor if you feel uneasy about treatment that is being suggested.

5. Avoid getting tired.
You can't see everything you would like without becoming exhausted. Take time out to rest.

All these ideas are ways of looking at — and getting involved in — the world around you. Politics, history, news stories, ecology, natural disasters, travel — all connect you to the world and touch you somehow. Which has the deepest influence on your view of the world? Use that organizing theme to begin thinking about assets, liabilities, resources, and what you can do on a global level. Then look at another angle, and see what it yields. The world leaves ample room for involvement!

Universe

If there are many ways of looking at the world, there are even more windows into the universe. Science, imagination, faith, even your personal identity can connect you to the cosmos. Do you read science fiction? It becomes more fantastic all the time. It has to, because some of the fantastic things written in older science fiction have now become realities. Communication and transportation between planets is no longer amazing. Presumably there are endless galaxies yet to be discovered. Everything that happens in the universal system has an effect on you. For one thing, your tax dollars pay for the men and machines to make exploratory trips. Scientific discoveries have already impacted our lives and will do so even more in the future. Some of the recent understanding about calcium metabolism has come about from studying people in zero gravity situations. How much have you read about developments in science? What would you like to know more about? One publication that contains brief reports on current research in a readable style is *Science News*, which is published weekly. You can subscribe by writing to Science Service, Inc., 1719 N Street, N.W., Washington, D.C., 20036, or you can read it at the library.

Living Systems Inventory

Universe

Assets	Liabilities	Resources

What I Can Do

Science is one tool for exploring the riches the universe has to offer; faith is another. Some people would argue that beliefs belong in the inner systems, in the brain, where thoughts are formed. It is included here because my belief is that there is a powerful being greater than myself, greater than the universe, and I call him God. What are your beliefs?

Who are you? Your identity is part of the fabric of this universe. You have a name and certain roles to play in life. You are genetically coded to look a certain way. You may be coded to have certain diseases. Some of your behavior may be the result of genetic coding, although you can train yourself to behave differently. What tells who you are? You, this complex person whose life depends upon the functioning of internal systems? You, who have somehow survived for more than half a century as part of many larger systems? Take time to think about your beliefs about yourself, your spirituality, and the universe. Then look for assets and liabilities. What facts, discoveries, or beliefs have made your life better? Which have not? Enter these into the Living Systems Inventory, *Universe*. Make room for science, faith, your identity, whatever helps the universe make sense to you. These directions are more open than in other sections because the universe, more than any other system, is what you make of it.

Taking Stock

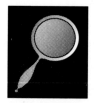
In order to organize all of these thoughts, you'll want to fill in the Master Living Systems Inventory on pages 216 and 217 so you can see what your overall assets and liabilities look like. This exercise gives you a chance to review the individual inventories you've completed so far, and to pull out ideas you'd like to hold on to, even explore further. You might begin by looking over your inventories on inner system, self, family, and friends from Chapters 1 and 2. Then you can come back to the inventories in this chapter on community, state, nation, world, and universe. You'll see that the master inventory begins with the broadest system — universe — and becomes gradually more focused, ending with yourself. Under "Myself: Outer Network" you have a chance to consider yourself in terms of work and social life; under "Myself: Inner System" you can consider your physical, emotional, and spiritual well-being. Fill things out in any order you like. Ideally, you'll see all these systems come together into a comprehensive picture of your unique living system as you fill out the master inventory.

Please take plenty of time for this. As you write, you may find that new issues and perspectives come into focus. That's perfectly all right; in fact, it reminds you that your life story isn't fixed, but continually evolving. Chances are you won't find room for everything on one chart. Let yourself be creative and open-minded in what you include. The process of selecting an item or two from each category may help you recognize priorities.

Completing your inventory will probably bring forth some feelings of sorrow, but hopefully some gladness, too. It involves a whole life review. When you are through, you should have a new perspective on where you are now and how you want the rest of your life to be. You can then start taking action to make it happen.

The next main section, "Achieving Your Goals," will help you translate the ideas in your Master Living Systems Inventory into concrete steps for action.

Sue

Sue's experience may help you get started. First of all, Sue did her inventory in pencil because she found that as she wrote, her beliefs became more clear, and revisions were needed. Even now she finds it useful to review and revise.

Take at look at the excerpts from Sue's Master Living Systems Inventory, which follows your inventory. The "Universe" section was important to Sue. She began by stating her belief in God and a divine plan. She was certain those beliefs were assets; some were resources. The hard part came when she had to find liabilities. She discovered that, although she believes in God, she sometimes feels distant from Him. "It seems like there's no one listening sometimes," she said. As she thought about that, she realized that it was not God who was distant, it was herself, moving away. That caused her to look at her own behaviors to see why she would remove herself from this source of comfort and guidance. She finally decided she wasn't focused enough to find direction, and that's what she wrote on her inventory under Liabilities. As you scan the roots on Nation and Myself (both Outer Network and Inner System) on Sue's chart, note how she translated both assets and liabilities into what she could do. Her inventory is personal, and your organization may not match it precisely. But try to look deeply into yourself in completing yours, and to reach far out into the world in effecting the changes you see a need for. It's up to you to reinforce the positive, and change the negative.

Achieving Your Goals

The final step toward achieving change is setting goals. It is best to be realistic, and focus on just a few goals at a time — more than that and your ambition might overwhelm you. If you start with two or three clear goals, you can set down practical steps you might take to achieve those goals, and can establish reasonable timeframes for each step. Once this is done, the question of "What can I do?" is given a real and manageable answer. Your project begins to look inspiring. The steps below can help you reach this stage.

Five Steps Towards Achieving Goals

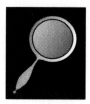

1. **Find the goals in your priorities and ambitions.**
   Look over your Master Living Systems Inventory. Chances are that you set many goals for yourself, some small and some very ambitious. The "What I Can Do" column is probably where you listed your initial goals. You'll also find goals suggested under the "Assets" column, where you

Master Living Systems Inventory

Systems	Assets	Liabilities	Resources	What I Can Do
Community				
Family				
Friends				
Myself: Outer Network				
Inner Systems				

Master Living Systems Inventory

Systems	Assets	Liabilities	Resources	What I Can Do
Universe				
World				
Nation				
State				

Sue's Master Living Systems Inventory

Systems	Assets	Liabilities	Resources	What I Can Do
Universe	I feel my life has a purpose, although I'm not always sure what it is.	Not always focused enough to find direction.	Myself, Heavenly Father, church, friends.	Meditate, pray, read scriptures. Visualization to help me focus. Change negative and fearful thoughts.
Nation	Freedom to do just about anything.	National debt/taxes; govermental corruption; Medicare less & less effective.	League of Women Voters, AARP, myself.	Prepare for election and vote; attend AARP meetings and support efforts regarding Medicare changes; use generic drugs and avoid expensive tests.
Community	Good low-income housing for elderly — pleasant place.	No public transportation; poor street lighting.	City council, businessmen's assoc., local newspaper.	Attend council meetings and express my concerns, or write letters to solicit support from BMA and medical.
Myself: Outer Network	Good at my job.	Dread retiring.	Community services, church, friends, Jake.	Assess my skills, examine unfulfilled desires — make a plan for rewarding volunteer work.
Inner System	Generally, good health.	Increasing deafness; cataract developing.	Myself, senior life programs at hospital, doctor.	Learn to read lips, investigate hearing aids; attend relevant classes at senior life; cataracts — make appointment with doctor.

listed things you might like to explore further, and under the "Liabilities" column, where you noted things you'd like to improve. Discover all the possible goals you set for yourself on the inventory, writing in more if you think of any.

2. Select a few goals from among the many to concentrate on.

You might do this by selecting one goal from each of the eight systems discussed on the Master Living Systems Inventory, and underlining it. Or you can just underline the half dozen that strike you as the most pressing. This is your target list of starting goals — but it's still too large to attack reasonably.

3. Write in the three top priority goals on the Goal Achievement Worksheet at the end of this chapter.

Limit yourself to three goals for the initial exercise, or even fewer if you like. You can always come back to include more, once you have achieved glorious success with these first goals. Write the name of the system that will benefit — such as community, or friends — on the top line for each listing, and the goal itself on the second line. Select these goals from your list of underlined goals, and be as ambitious as you like in the selection. It is in writing down practical steps that you'll need to be realistic.

4. Consider the precise steps you'll need to take to achieve your goals, and write them down with expected dates of completion.

Write only things you think you'll really do. Set only dates you think you can meet. (One exception is goals that involve a new way of looking at yourself or the world; start those as soon as you think of them!) If, through this process, a specific goal starts to look unattainable, select a new one you think you can reach. Perhaps you can simply modify the original goal. Remember, the goal in goal-setting is personal reward as well as world improvement!

5. Set yourself up to succeed.

Expect that you will accomplish the goals you set to the best of your ability in the time given. Be tolerant of yourself when you fall short. Pick yourself up after failure and try again.

It might help you, before beginning your worksheet on the next page, to see how Sue filled out part of her Goal Achievement Worksheet

---

Sue's Goal Achievement Worksheet

System: *World*
Goal: *Help preserve fragile ecosystem*
Steps to Take: *Call city for recyclng pick-up.*   By: *Tomorrow*
                  Conserve water.   *Now*
                  Plant trees.   *This autumn*

System: *. Community*
Goal: *Better street lighting*
Steps to Take: *Call city council, find out date of*   By: *Tomorrow*
                     next meeting.
                  Write letter to newspaper.   *Friday*
                  Attend city council meeting.   *?*

System: *Family*
Goal: *Be a better sister to Jake*
Steps to Take: *Stop nagging about his smoking.*   By: *Today*
                  Express desire to see him more,   *Next week*
                     invite him for a walk.

You have a built-in urge to be perfect. Over your lifetime you may have accomplished many things to near perfection. Very likely you have failed at some tasks. That is as it should be. The hallmark of a productive person is that she has not been daunted by failure. In fact, she has failed her way to success. Be prepared to succeed, and recognize failures as steps in the ladder. Keep your goals with you as you go through each day, and you won't lose sight of the top of the ladder. The world is a better place for your having been here. Even small actions count up to big contributions

References

Hollender, J. (1990) *How to Make the World a Better Place.* New York: William Morrow and Company, Inc.

Goal Achievement Worksheet

System: _____

Goal: _____

Steps to Take:_____   By: _____

_____   _____

_____   _____

System: _____

Goal: _____

Steps to Take:_____   By: _____

_____   _____

_____   _____

System: _____

Goal: _____

Steps to Take:_____   By: _____

_____   _____

_____   _____

System: _____

Goal: _____

Steps to Take:_____   By: _____

_____   _____

_____   _____

10

The Closing Chord

Although this chapter is supposed to be about the ending of life, it is really about living; for grief and dealing with death are a part of every human life. What this chapter offers is help in anticipating death, understanding how to live with its inevitability, and growing from the experience. It's for you, *now*.

The saddest woman I ever knew was a woman who claimed she had no faith. Rikha was a talented woman. She was a concert pianist and a fine teacher. Well-read and intelligent, she could converse knowledgeably about world events. She was a pretty woman, too, with snapping black eyes and graying black hair artistically twisted to the back of her small head. But Rikha, at 63, was unhappy.

When her husband died, Rikha's black eyes lost their sparkle. Something inside of Rikha faded. She said to me one day, "I wish I could believe in something. Sigmund is gone, he is absent, there is no Sigmund anymore."

"What do you think happens to people when they die?" I asked.

"Nothing happens to them. That's the end of it. Cremate them and dump the ashes, there's nothing more."

No matter how much Rikha wanted to believe in some kind of God or power larger than herself, she was unable to do it. She was unable to find solace in a life lived for its own beauty, either. The believing part of her was dead. She didn't even believe in herself as having any power. Life was a physical, biological event that ran its course with no meaning and then ended. The idea of soul or spirit was so foreign to her that she could not grasp it. I think this is why Rikha was sad.

Faith

What you believe is unique, and may be very different from your neighbor's belief, or mine.

In my view, emotional pain suggests the presence of a spirit, or soul, if you will. If life were simply a biological event, why would there be this innate striving to stay alive, to excel, to be happy? It cannot be satisfactorily explained on the basis of neurochemical theories. Albert Schweitzer, a German medical missionary who lived in the first half of this century, said: "No ray of sunlight is ever lost, but the green which it awakes into existence needs time to sprout, and it is not always granted to the sower to see the harvest. All work that is worth anything is done in faith."

One of America's first statesmen and a signer of the constitution, William Penn, said in his succinct and pithy way, "The truest end of life is to know the life that never ends." And Johann Wolfgang von Goethe, 18th century philosopher, amplified Penn's thought: "When a man is as old as I am, he is bound occasionally to think about death. In my case this thought leaves me in perfect peace, for I have a firm conviction that our spirit is a being indestructible by nature. It works on from eternity; it is like the sun which only seems to set, but in truth never sets but shines on unceasingly."

Your faith may not be phrased in terms of "God," "spirit," or "soul." It may follow the teachings of an organized religion, or it may be entirely of your own formation. Whatever shape it has, it can be an enormous support. Throughout this chapter try looking inside yourself to find the expression of faith that makes sense to you. If these beliefs come from your own hopes and experiences, they will enable you to face every experience — including death — with hope.

Everyone thinks about death. In times of war, children think about death a good deal more than is good for them. When you are ill, you are apt to let your thoughts dwell on the possibility of death. After the age of 60, you begin to think of it more often, for at that age you have already experienced the loss of friends and family members. You may not have paid much attention to the obituary column before, but now you find yourself searching for familiar names. When none of the people whose names are listed are known to you, you may sigh and think, "Thank goodness."

You have been preparing for death all of your life, even though this preparation may not have been present in your conscious mind. Since you have become older, and I hope since you have been reading this book, you have made other preparations. At this time, a summing up is in order so that you can see if you have left anything undone. Preparation for life and its inevitable end depends upon faith — your faith in yourself, and in the universal order of things.

Faith is personal and intimate. Someone else cannot give you faith, nor can you give it to another. Faith can be inspired by certain events or the behaviors and attitudes of someone you admire, but eventually it can only come from within you. My husband, Walt, tells about World War II.

"The chaplain of our unit held religious services every Sunday morning. Usually there weren't many there — just me and few others. After the invasion into Normandy, there were so many in attendance that the services had to be moved into the mess hall."

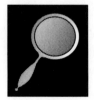 How did your faith develop? What does your faith tell you about life and death? At this time it would be very useful for you to write about your faith — tell what you believe and how you came to believe it. To start, think about the ways in which your faith helps you to make preparations for the summing up of your life on earth. Use this space, or a blank piece of paper, or your journal to pour your heart out. You can use the suggested phrases to

begin, or ignore them. No one need see it unless you want them to. If someone is interested in this book, buy them a new one and keep this one to yourself.

My Faith
I believe

I hope

I hold on to

I anticipate

Defining your faith can help you focus on life from a meaningful perspective. You're going to leave some things behind when you go, and so now is the time to think about what and how you want to do that.

Preparing a Personal Legacy

By now you will have prepared a will or revocable trust document, and your durable power of attorney has been taken care of. The legacy I'm thinking of now is you. What do you want to leave the world that will speak of the person, the intellect, and the spirit that is beautifully and uniquely you? How do you preserve the essence of your personality? How can you give others the benefit of your experience and wisdom when you are no longer here?

What I have in mind are the things you create. These include your personal history, which you may have composed in an earlier chapter; your art; your music; your writing. Perhaps you make quilts or braid rugs. All of these things speak of you. A Mozart symphony makes Mozart, the man, real. The painting my mother did at age 85 brings her smile and her energy into the present. The violins my son made speak to me with his voice. What do you have that activates the memories of people you have known? Do you have letters from long ago? Pictures?

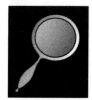 The form on the next page will help you assess what you have already done and discover what you might yet do to leave your personal legacy. Take your time, be thoughtful, and think about the people for whom you are leaving this legacy. It will probably not be just your family. There will be broader impact than that. Stradivarius never had an idea that his instruments would be sought after by people all over the world hundreds of years after his death. I doubt if Flannery O'Connor expected that the letters she wrote to her friends would be put into a book to be read by millions of people. Instead of asking yourself, "Who would ever want that?" tell yourself, "When my great- grandchildren see this, they will begin to know me, even if they have never seen me in person."

At some points you may feel stuck, unable to fill in all the blanks. It takes time and thought to do this kind of thing. You may need to set it aside and let your brain do the work for you as you engage in some other activity. When you come back to it, you will

My Personal Legacy

Journal: I have kept a journal, and it may be found _____

_____

Talents and Skills: The evidence of my special talents may be seen _____

_____

_____

_____

   (I have written, drawn, painted, sculpted, performed, and so forth.)

As I review my life, I see that I leave behind_____

_____

_____

_____

   (Think beyond material assets like a house, a car, or a bank account.)

New skills I am working on now include _____

_____

_____

I expect from these new skills there will be _____

_____

_____

Memorable Times: The memorable times of sharing my experiences verbally with others include _____

_____

_____

   (You could tell some memories to a tape recorder, too.)

I look forward to sharing _____

_____

_____

find that what you wanted to say is right there, ready to be written. It's interesting that in order to think about death, you have to think a great deal about life.

Funeral Planning

Planning your own funeral may sound morbid, but it can be a very rewarding project. The section that follows will lead you through some basic steps in funeral planning, should you choose to consider them. The project is entirely optional. Sometimes it can ease fear and bring peace. It's another way of feeling in control, and it reminds you of the day-to-day normal sequence of progression through life. On the other hand, it could be depressing. If so, feel free not to worry about it — that's your privilege. Sometimes it's good for the family to have concrete things to do and to focus on in the aftermath of a death. The funeral is partially a ritual for them, after all. If you feel that having a part in the ritual would help you cope *now* with the thought of your own death, consider the following guidelines.

The Purpose of a Funeral

The deathbed scene, with loved ones hovering tearfully nearby, is not the place for funeral planning. Gasping out instructions to a distressed spouse adds tension to an already highly stressful moment. Any energy available in those precious last hours should be for being together, silently if you like, and for saying goodbye. Funeral plans should be thought out, discussed, and recorded during a time when you feel strong and capable. Now would be a good time.

Who is the funeral for? Is it for you? Or is it for those who stay behind? I think it is for both. I'd like to share an image that brings me solace; perhaps you have your own that captures your beliefs about death. Suppose you are on a long trip with your family and friends. You are going to a beautiful island where the climate is moderate and food is plentiful. You expect to have a pleasant and peaceful time there. Some of the family is already there, waiting to greet you. It has been decided that you will take a train across the land and then charter a boat to get to the island. There is some risk involved in this journey, but you'll be together, and for the most part it appears that it will be quite enjoyable. When you have traveled about half the distance, you receive a telegram telling you of an emergency that will require your presence on the island much sooner than you had planned. The only thing to do is to get off the train at the next stop and catch a plane. You hate to leave family and friends, and they are sad at the thought of making the journey without you, but so it must be. Of course, there are arrangements to be discussed and plans to be made, for things will be different without you. There are certain things you want done to ensure safety for the family. Once the plans are made, you can relax and enjoy the last few hours before you have to leave them.

That's what a funeral plan does, in my view. You want the funeral to be something that will further strengthen the bond with your loved ones. Admittedly it is a ritual, but an important one, for it is the passage by which your family can begin the new life without your presence. Psychologist Therese Rando describes the benefits of funerary rituals, and notes that similar rituals are observed in various ways in nearly every culture. For instance (adapted from her book, *Grief, Dying, and Death*):

1. The funeral provides social support for those who are grieving, bringing together relatives and friends who communicate their care and their intention to provide comfort and support.

2. The ceremony or ritual explains the reason for and meaning of death.

3. Often there is a viewing of the body, whether at the funeral or in another place before the funeral.

4. There is usually a procession, which allows people to display their grief publicly. It usually concludes the funeral by ending at the place of burial.

5. Some kind of sanitary disposition of the body is carried out, such as burial, entombment, or cremation.

6. Funerals require material expenditure, even if you have arranged for a prepaid funeral. This enables the grievers to communicate their loss to society and support this sentiment with tangible, measurable means.

The ritual of the funeral has been misunderstood, and those whose profession it is to carry out these functions have been severely criticized at times. Isn't it odd that there are specialists for the ritual of marriage, which is also a passage to a new life, but rarely are they criticized. In fact, people are prepared to pay two or three times as much for a wedding as they do for a funeral.

Rituals serve to defuse anxiety and mobilize a network of support for the coming time of adjustment. The funeral serves three long-term purposes for the person who has died and for those who are grieving. First, for the grieving person the funeral affirms separation from the loved one. Second, it realizes the transition into a state of being which does not include the loved one. And third, it facilitates the incorporation into a social group in this changed state. In other words, your place in society is no longer that of Charlie Brown's wife, or of Sally Jones' father, you are now just you, in the beginning phases of forming a new social identity.

For the deceased person, the funeral symbolically removes his physical presence from his family and friends. It also serves as a passage or transition into the state of death. The reality of his death is acknowledged and affirmed as he is left in the land of the dead. Most importantly, the funeral validates the life of the deceased by giving testimony to the fact that a life has been lived. There is evidence that doing away with the funeral results in unresolved guilt, pent-up anger, and the sorrow of half-finished relationships. Without the ritual for openly and shamelessly expressing the normal emotions of grief, other outlets which are less therapeutic will be used, such as illness or aggressive and hostile acts against society.

Gerald

Gerald is an angry man. His father died when Gerald was a young man, and the family decided not to have any kind of funeral or service. The body was cremated and the ashes were sent to Gerald's home. Gerald stuck the package on a closet shelf, telling himself it was better to just forget all about it. Over the years he developed a series of stress-related illnesses. He became cantankerous and taciturn. When he required surgery for a bleeding ulcer, he was an obstinate, angry patient. A nurse, puzzled by his behavior, decided to confront him.

Nurse: (*while removing the blood pressure cuff*) You seem to be upset.

Gerald: Damn right, you would be, too, if you had your belly cut, and couldn't even get decent care.

Nurse: Sounds like you feel neglected and abused.

Gerald: Well, maybe not abused, but neglected for sure.

Nurse: I'm wondering if you weren't pretty angry before you got sick.

Gerald: Things sure haven't gone right for me the last couple of years.

Nurse: Tell me about it.

Then Gerald began to talk about his business trials, and family problems, and finally his father's death.

Nurse: That's tough, to lose your dad.

Gerald: I didn't know it would be so tough. It's like something gnawing at me, you know, something that never goes away.

Nurse: Was the funeral difficult for you?

Gerald: (*with a tear creeping down his face*) There wasn't any funeral. We all thought it was better not to make too much of it.

Nurse: No wonder you feel anxious and unfinished. Maybe that's what chewed the big hole in your stomach.

As they talked further, Gerald came up with the idea that he could do something to finish the whole business of his dad's death. He decided to get his brothers and sisters together for an informal memorial. Some were reluctant, but finally agreed.

They shared memories of both good times and bad times. They were able to talk about the feelings of guilt and anger and to support each other. Then they decided to purchase a tree for the city's downtown beautification project. That way they would have a living memorial to their father.

Gerald's health improved after that, and he felt less anxious and angry. His wife and children noticed the improvement and stopped avoiding him. Gerald needed a ritual to complete the physical separation from his father.

Planning the Details

There are valid reasons for whatever ritual you choose. Cremation and memorial services held after the burial are variations on traditional funeral services. Cremation that is done without any kind of memorial service should not be chosen as a way of avoiding the pain of grief. Bypassing the ritual delays the completion of grief. In fact, in a large-scale study of widows and widowers done in 1976, the results showed that those who participated in a traditional funeral (which included viewing the body and having friends and relatives present) had fewer adjustment problems than those who had less than the traditional funeral. Those who did not view the body or who had arranged for immediate disposition of the body were reported as having had the greatest hostility following death, the greatest increase in consumption of alcohol, tranquilizers, and sedatives, the greatest increase in tension and anxiety, the lowest positive recall of the deceased, and greater problems in adjustment to death. This was particularly true in male respondents.

Assuming that you are going to choose a traditional funeral, even though it may include cremation, there are important decisions you can make now.

Choosing a Funeral Director

Again, this is optional, as are all of the suggestions about funeral planning. Choose the parts you would like to do and leave the rest out.

In most states, there are regulations about the disposal of a body. Your children can't bury you under your favorite apple tree. Unless you are going to be buried within 24 hours, you will have to be embalmed. You have probably attended a few funerals in your lifetime and have some idea about what kind of work various directors do. I know of one establishment that will arrange the body in a sitting position. Another does a Hollywood job of makeup. Neither of those appeal to me, but they fill the needs of others. Choose the one that gives the kind of funeral you have felt good about in the past. Do some comparison shopping — visit the places you are interested in and get a feel for the attitudes of the staff. You can prepay for your funeral, or you can set aside money in some interest-gathering account and designate it for that purpose. Remember that the funeral may cost a little more 10 years from now.

Choosing a Burial Place

Some caution should be exercised here. The lovely place out in the country on top of a hill may seem idyllic to you. Unfortunately, it may be inaccessible to family and friends. Some people rarely visit cemeteries, while others derive great comfort from the ritual of visiting the grave site. No one can predict how they will feel about it until the time comes. You may not have enjoyed visiting a grave site in the past, but every death is different. Your children think they know how they will feel, but things may turn out in an entirely different way. One thing you can't anticipate is how you'll handle death.

Selecting a Casket, Urn, and Location of Funeral

You really can't choose a specific casket, but you can decide in general what you'd like and specify a price range. You don't even have to have a casket in most states. If your grandson, the carpenter, wants to build a box, there's no reason why he can't. Stories abound about people who have made their own box well in advance. (An interesting idea, one which is not likely to become popular, I think.) Do think about whether you really want to make decisions in this much detail. There is therapeutic value for the family in selecting a casket. It is the last caring act they can do for you. It is symbolic of tucking you in and saying "good night." Maybe you should let them have that privilege. This may be true of other aspects of your funeral planning, too. It depends upon your relationship with family members, and how great the importance of doing your own deciding is with regard to the funeral.

Planning the Service

This is the area in which most people have an interest in making directives. Depending upon your religion or beliefs, it is likely that someone is going to give a talk about you. Now you have to decide if that is what you want. Some don't. Some prefer to have funeral talks about religion, about the doctrines and principles relating to death and the hereafter. Some want both. In any event, you might like to make suggestions about who would give these talks, and who will read the obituary. If the talks are going to be about you, do you want them to be serious and profound, or would you like a bit of humor, something that shows you were a fallible human being?

When Beatrice died, her daughters knew she had left written instructions about the funeral. Beatrice wrote, "I don't want sadness. You can cry, that's healthy, but don't carry on about how terrible it was that I died. I made a lot of mistakes in my life. I hope I did a few good things. Whoever (your choice) talks about me at the funeral, tell them not to make me look better than I am. A little laughter at some of the funny things would be a relief. For example, do you remember the times we had to get out and push the old Model T Ford up the hill to the lake? If you do, you'll remember how we fell in a mud puddle and Janie said, "Daddy, Mommy's made an old bad mess!" I hope I haven't made an "old bad mess" out of my life, I don't think I have, but please just try to remember me as I really am, not as some glorified creature nobody will recognize."

Music is often an important part of the funeral service. It is good to make your favorite selections known. There has to be leeway for your family to choose something, too, but they will feel good about having the music you had wanted. My mother's funeral was all music because we are all musicians. To us, the music spoke a stronger message than anyone could have given verbally. We don't know if she wanted it that way because she never told us, but she loved music. My father, on the other hand, gave instructions as he lay dying. It meant a great deal to us to include in his service the person he most wanted to have sing his favorite song. This is a gift you give your family, just as the casket may be their gift to you. The message in the music is a way of saying goodbye after your voice has been stilled.

While you're planning the service, don't forget the graveside ritual. Often the grave is dedicated, and you may have feelings about whom you would like to have give that dedication. There can be other rituals, too, even some of your own making. My sister gave all the little great-grandchildren pennies to toss into the grave. I don't remember what the significance of that was, but I do know that they remember the part they had to play, and it was important to them. You can have whatever you want, including a brass band if you so desire, but you need to write it down, make it known.

Sometimes a dinner or other gathering takes place when all the rituals are completed. These gatherings are important for the family to be able to integrate in their new roles. Feeding people and being fed are interactive nurturing tasks. Those who are feeding are saying, "You're empty now, let us fill the aching spot," while those being fed accept this symbolic replacement. Even aside from symbolism, eating stimulates the release of endorphins that help ease the pain of loss. You can't plan the dinner, but you might want to make suggestions about it. For example, one woman has directed that games be played so that the children will remember the experience in a happy way.

Here is a funeral plan worked out by a friend of mine. She calls it a "graduation exercise" because she thinks that's what death is — a graduation from the school of earthly life to a life that is unimaginably better. You could call it something else, if you like.

Creating Your Goodbye

Allow your own tastes, style, and desires to show in your plan for the graduation exercise. Give yourself permission to have control over the end and to think about it now. This is the metaphor one woman chose, along with the written directions she completed as a soothing exercise. Annie died of cancer at age 70. She never married, and so it was a niece who carried out her wishes.

Graduation Exercise

1. When the time comes for me to graduate from this life, I have arranged with the following funeral home for their services:
   Andrews Mortuary
   912 Walnut Way
   467-5200

These services may be paid for with money from a CD held in trust for you at Third National Bank in Oklahoma City.

2. For my final resting place I have chosen Lakeview Cemetery. I thought this would be convenient for you, but if you prefer another place, I will be happy with your choice. There is more than enough in the CD to pay for this, too.

3. Here is an outline of the graduation service. Feel free to add anything or anyone if you wish.

Prayer: by Pastor Williamson of the Prince of Glory Lutheran Church. I taught him in high school, and he still comes to see me once in a while. He's been a good friend.

Hymns: *Abide With Me*
Oh My Father

Scripture: John 3:16. If Iva Fields is still around, ask her to read. She has such a nice voice, and she's been my closest friend for 40 years. I think she can do this without crying because she doesn't think death is sad anymore than I do.

Special Music: Dan Wetherby sang at your wedding, and I've known him since he was a toddler. I'd love it if he could sing *I Know That My Redeemer Lives*. This next one probably sounds a little strange for a funeral, but there's an old, old song my father used to sing that I'd like. It needs a bass voice, though, and right now I don't know any basses. See what you can do about getting someone to sing *Old Man River*.

Talks: Do you think Randy could do it? I know it's hard for family members, but he's just been so dear to me, a really special grandnephew. Tell him not to get too serious. We had some good laughs. Tell him he doesn't need to make people bawl.

Then, of course, I'd like Bishop Brown, or whoever is Bishop at the time of my graduation, to speak. Some uplifting thoughts about life and death and the hereafter, whatever he wants.

Obituary: I have written my own, which may seem vain, but I know better than anyone what my life was like. Since I will be unable to read it, you could, or you could ask someone who's still alive who knew me. No strangers, please, they always want to make the dead person sound like a saint, which I wasn't.

More Special Music: If you can, round up a string trio or quartet that would make me sit up and take notice. Interesting mental picture. I had a good time making music in my life, seems fitting for my graduation.

Closing Prayer: Ask the Relief Society president. I hope it's still Marie Quentan. She helped me laugh at myself when I was depressed about the cancer. Give her a big hug for me.

Dedication of the Grave: Bishop Brown can do this, too.

My Valedictory Address: Isn't this fun? I always wanted to be the valedictorian, but I missed it by a fraction.

Valediction means a farewell, and it's given at school graduations by the highest ranking student. It implies that the farewell is not of a permanent nature, the speaker is going on to bigger and better things, and exhorts his classmates to do the same. I don't know what my rank is at this point, but it's my funeral so I can be valedictorian if I want.

It seems to me, looking back, that life has been very short, but I remember how long it was when I was going through it. There were a lot of hard lessons and a few great disappointments. When I was young, I pictured myself married to a good-looking, solid man. I expected to have five or six children. There wasn't much else I wanted to do, I thought. Well, it wasn't to be. I don't know why, but I never met anyone I liked well enough to marry. I fell in love a few times, but there wasn't enough liking to make me want to live with a man for 50 years. I did have the children, though, not five or six, but several hundred. Teaching was not a career I chose, it chose me. It didn't pay very well, and I worked more hours than I really wanted to, but there was something about it that held me. I guess it was seeing those oddly dressed, unfocused, often rude, and always confused young people unfold, wake up, and blossom into remarkably astute and likeable adults. Some of them are still my good friends.

The school I attended was not in a classroom per se. It was on the streets, in the theaters, in my apartment alone at night, in the homes of friends, and certainly in church and in the hospitals. They, whoever "they" are, call it the school of hard knocks. There are hard knocks, it's true, but this school is more like following a stream to it's source. You have to climb some, you fall down a little, but it's exciting. The challenge is to grow stronger along the way, and the reward is to finally reach the source and be welcomed just as you are, scars and all.

I don't have anything more to say. I've completed my journey, and I'm eager to go on. I love you, dear niece, as if you were my own birth child. It's time for me to go, but I'll look forward to seeing you there in 30 or 40 years. Just follow the stream upward.

Your Life Story

 Now the one remaining part of your goodbye is the writing of your obituary. Writing your obituary, like all of the other planning you've been doing, is a way to get in touch with your current life and yourself as a unique person. As you write, think about all the things you can still do.

Don't worry about the space limitations imposed by a newspaper. Set aside fears of sounding vain or foolish. You don't need a high governmental position to have an interesting life. Your life *is* interesting. No other person has had a life like yours. I have never read a boring obituary. Bear in mind that it is your life as you remember it, not how someone who only knew you for a portion of it sees it.

The point of writing an obituary is to focus on your *life*. What have you done that you can feel good about? What can you still do? You might write something just for yourself, regardless of whether it will wind up in a newspaper.

Give up all concerns about spelling, grammar, and other hindrances to free expression. Just write. Start with your name, the date of your birth, and where you were born. Tell who your parents were and where you went to school. Talk about all the things you'd like the world to know. Describe the events and activities that are important to you, that give others a picture of who you are. Do a visualization of yourself as a young person. What were your goals? Which ones were met? Which new ones appeared as you became more mature? What have you discovered about yourself? Are there unsolved mysteries? What goals do you have now for the rest of your life? What can you still explore?

It doesn't matter if you fill 10 pages, just keep writing. Then put it away for a week. When you get it out again, you can begin to edit. Some of the things you told may not be exactly what you want remembered, or in the newspaper. Cut those things out. I mean literally, with the scissors, or delete them on the computer. When you've finished cutting, paste together what's left. Once again, set it aside for a couple of days. The next time you look at it, you will see other things you want to change. Repeat this process until you have exactly what you want. You will probably cut out quite a few things, and maybe add some. When you're finished with it, put it away until some noteworthy event occurs, and then go back and see if you want to add to it. Keep doing this. It may be years between updates, or it may be more frequent.

Eventually, you may want to concern yourself with length — especially if yours is the obituary you'd like published. If so, call the editor of the local and regional section of the newspaper and ask what the acceptable length for an obituary is. She may tell you that she has a form to be filled out from which a staff writer will create your obituary. Never mind that, they'll print what you write if you keep the length within their guidelines. If she tells you column inches, ask for number of words. That's all the interaction you'll have with the newspaper. Go over your obituary and edit out unnecessary adjectives, ands, buts, thats, and whiches. Count the words and edit again. Be sure that your responsible person knows where to find it. Most people find that writing their own obituary is a uniquely healing task. When you have finished writing, you will probably have a mixture of feelings — sadness, relief, pride. Now that it's written, you need to get back to the here and now. Use the following questions for examining your opportunities for growth now.

Here-and-Now Reflection

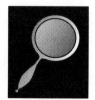

1. In what ways would I still like to change and grow?
2. What am I most proud of in my life? (For example, perhaps the greatest pride has been in being a parent. Use that answer as the springboard for the following questions.)
3. How can I become more involved in that aspect of my life now?
4. How can I use this pride to become involved at a community level?
5. Are there failures I can correct by service to someone now?

6. What things have I meant to do and not done that I can still do now?

Act now on these things — your life story isn't over. This is also a good time to go over the Advance Preparation Checklist that follows and tidy up unfinished business.

Advance Preparation Checklist

❑ Will or Revocable Trust.
❑ Living Will or Durable Power of Attorney for Health Care.
❑ Copies of the above to responsible family member.
❑ Personal history written.
❑ Family notified about location of important papers, such as insurance documents, bank accounts, and so forth.
❑ Funeral planned (optional).
❑ Funeral plans discussed with family or clergy.
❑ Burial arrangements made and paid for (optional).
❑ Amends made to those I may have offended.
❑ Reconciliation with alienated loved ones.
❑ Gratitude and appreciation expressed to those who have affected my life in a positive way.
❑ Special gifts of personal property given.
❑ Dependent members of the family arranged for.
❑ Religious concerns resolved.
❑ Personal legacies completed or in progress.
❑ Letters written to those who will be remaining behind.
❑ Personal effects sorted and organized.
❑ Business affairs in order.
❑ Transfer of title to my home (in the absence of revocable trust).
❑ Disposition of vehicles arranged for.
❑ At peace and ready to go, but eager to keep living.

When You Are Not the First To Go

Does it seem that this chapter goes about things in the wrong order? It does, but for a purpose. It's easier to deal with someone else's death if you have come to terms with your own. Every death is accompanied by grief. There is no way around it. You can only go through it. Those who try to avoid it or deny it are only prolonging it. You just need to know up front that you will mourn for at least a year, and after that you will mourn on special days.

Letting Yourself Grieve

Grief, mourning, bereavement — whatever you choose to call it — is not a bad thing. It is painful, but there is value in it. Grief is an intimate experience that offers you the opportunity to grow. Reactions to grief are as varied as there are people who experience them. Grief is physical, emotional, and social.

Immediately after the death of a loved one you may feel numb, unfeeling, unable to take it in. During this time you may experience agitation, sorrow, and anger. At times you may pace the floor, walk through the rooms of your home, or go shopping with no purpose. It is as if you are searching for something. At other times you may feel heavy and weak, lapsing into inactivity for hours at a time. Physically, your heart may beat faster, and you will have increased cortisol and catecholamines in your bloodstream. You will probably find yourself saying things such as, "I don't believe it," "It just can't be true," "It doesn't seem like he could really be gone." This acute phase may last for minutes, hours, or weeks.

Then comes despair. Bodily distress, which comes in waves, may include tightness in the throat, a feeling of suffocation and panic, weakness, insomnia or sleeping too much, and a feeling of emptiness or pain in the stomach and abdomen. You may experience loss of appetite resulting in loss of weight, or you may want to eat all the time and gain a lot of weight. At times you will feel angry toward your loved one. At other times you may be overwhelmed with guilt, questioning things you said or failed to say, regretting something you did, perhaps. You wonder if you will feel terrible forever.

Grief has a profound effect on the immune system. Studies in the United States and in Australia have shown that individuals in grief have impaired function of T-lymphocytes. Hormonal irregularities have been demonstrated. These changes can make you susceptible to illness. Your immune system may not be able to fight off bacterial or viral infection. Grief is stress. Loss creates internal disequilibrium. It is a great strain to try to regain balance internally as well as socially. The behaviors you have used in the past to handle stress often seem useless for handling grief. You are being asked to reconcile yourself to an event that can't be changed. You have no control over death.

If you are willing to experience the pain fully without stopping it with drugs or chronic depression, the pain will lessen bit by bit, month by month. For a long time the pain will come surging back on anniversaries and other special occasions, and it will be just as intense as it was at the beginning. There is hope, some sunshine ahead. Each month the pain will be less until finally it becomes a poignant sadness, integrated into your personality, either adaptively or maladaptively. Ultimately the most adaptive response is to celebrate the life which ended and to begin to create a new life from the wisdom gleaned from suffering.

Give yourself a year to get through the grief. During that time, table all major decisions. Stay put, don't move to a different place if you can possibly avoid it. Stay in your job, keep doing your volunteer work, and maintain relationships, no matter how hard it is. "Dying is hard work," said my friend when her father was dying. I say grieving is hard work, too. There are three parts to doing grief work: resolving anger, learning to receive love, and letting go of guilt. While you're doing this work, you need to nurture yourself by taking care of basic needs.

Taking Care of Your Basic Needs

There are healthy and unhealthy ways to meet your needs. Among the healthy ways is keeping your faith alive and growing. There is meaning in life, and there are reasons to continue living — you may just have to search for that meaning. Reaching out to people and getting involved in new activities are healthy ways of coping, when you're ready for them. But you must avoid turning to unhealthy, destructive ways of coping. You can damage your health and your emotional stability by over- or undereating, overworking, and overdependence on others.

Need for Food

Think back to childhood days. Remember the tasty dishes your mother prepared for you at special times or just because she knew you liked them? That nice coconut cream pie she used to make may be just the thing to spark your appetite. Never mind for the moment that it is high in fat and cholesterol. You're not going to pig out on pie every day. Think of it as first-aid medicine you're going to take just to get you over the worst pain. Then you will feel better enough to be rational about food, and eat the healthier medicine your body will need. This applies whether you have lost interest in food or whether you have suddenly gained a desire to eat everything in sight. The following suggestions have helped some people get through the problem-eating period.

Mealtime Guidelines

1. *Set the table attractively for your meal.* Use dishes and silverware that you especially like. You may not want to do this. You may resist it with all your might, but do it anyway. Just say to yourself, "This is good for me." If you feel that you want to stand at the refrigerator and stuff yourself, set the table especially nicely and make yourself sit. If you don't want to eat at all, this may inspire you to get at least minimal nourishment.

2. *Prepare just enough food so there are no leftovers.* Those small portions stashed in the refrigerator are bad for stand-up, desperation eating. That kind of snacking is not good for either under- or overeaters. It builds a habit you'll wish you didn't have.

3. *Make sure you have food of three different colors on your plate.* For a while you may not feel like contending with nutritional concepts, but if you have three colors, you stand some chance of having a well-balanced meal. Of course, that doesn't mean three cupcakes with different-colored icings.

4. *Do whatever you have to do to make the meal enjoyable.* Include a favorite program or book, for instance. If you tend to overeat, remember that pairing eating with TV-watching can lead to more between-meals eating than is good for you. Make the meal enjoyable in

a way that will not build a bad habit. Many people can eat while reading and watching TV and have no problem. You know yourself; do what's right for you.

Need for Shelter

For most of us in this fast-paced world, shelter is more than a roof and walls. It is a place of beauty, warmth, and security. Many widowed persons have written to say that moving, which seemed a good idea at the time, turned out to be disastrous. Stay where you are if you can for a year.

For a time you may need to lower your expectations about the appearance of your home. If you are experiencing a low energy level, you may find it difficult to clean and cook and keep things as nice as you normally do.

Now is the time to develop a one-thing-at-a-time approach. Reject any thought of wholesale housecleaning. Do just one room, or one shelf, or dust one piece of furniture at a time. Adopt the same principle at work. Plan to accomplish just one task, using a larger block of time than usual. Your energy will return, you will work as quickly and effectively as you once did, but it takes time. It is best to defer any major redecorating until a year has passed. It is amazing how your ideas and color preferences can change during a period of grief.

Need for Love

Human beings of any age need love. It is necessary for life. I once knew a woman who had 50 cats. She had no person in the world to care for her — so she had 50 cats.

When you lose someone you love, you lose a piece of yourself. Many have described the feeling as having flesh forcibly torn from the body, leaving a dreadful wound. One man said it was like losing a million-dollar investment. Perhaps that is more accurate than you think. You invested a great deal in your beloved, and you received interest. Now it's like the bank closed. In time you will find that you can make new investments. In time you will realize that the original investment is still secure in your memories and your mature personality. In the meantime, you need nurturance.

You know what things comfort you, so make a list of them here.

_____

_____

_____

_____

Here are some ideas that have helped others who were grieving:

- *A warm bath.* If you like, scent it with your favorite aroma.
- *A daily schedule of exercise, alone or with a friend.* Walking, swimming, and biking are acceptable activities. Exercise makes you feel better for several reasons. If done consistently, biochemical changes occur in the body which tend to normal-

ize the adverse effects of grief. In that way, you are doing something to protect yourself from illness. The very act of going out and doing something physical is mentally invigorating.

- *Personal contact.* Giving love to others always results in a flow of love coming back. Volunteer work or spending more time with the family gives the opportunity to give love.
- *Writing a letter to the person who has died.* Tell him or her how you feel about being left. Reminisce about the good times you had together. Write about what you are going to do with your life now. (Keep this letter, for you will be writing again.)
- *A creative outlet.* Try an activity such as drawing, writing, or making something from yarn, cloth, or wood. Using your brain and your hand, for creation has a cathartic and energizing effect.

Nurturing yourself is a most important aid to comfortable, productive living. Grief is not a disease, but it is a painful life process. You can help yourself to grow and to become more truly your own person by caring for yourself. When you do that, you are better able to care for others. And you will make your progress through the grief process as damage-free as possible.

Dealing with Anger

There are certain rituals for the griever which help to face and resolve anger — a strong component of the grief process. The word "ritual" may summon visions of the macabre, but in reality everyone has certain rituals that give each day stability. Brushing your teeth is a ritual. Making the bed is a ritual. Hanging your tools up in a certain order is a ritual. When these things are left undone, you feel disorganized and incomplete. You are going to create some new rituals for dealing with anger. There are three types of rituals that can help you:

1. Act out.

Do something to vent your feelings. Vigorous exercise is one way, scrubbing floors is another. Working with clay, or taking up an aggressive activity such as darts or tennis would work. What could you do that would release some of the angry energy that keeps you tense and miserable? What has been a good active release in the past? Brainstorm in this space.

_____

_____

_____

_____

_____

2. Make feelings legitimate.

You need something that gives you permission to express feelings. You don't need to become analytical about why you feel the way you do — just know that people in grief feel anger. It's all right to be angry. You might write a letter expressing your anger. You could write a story about someone who is hurt and feels angry. In the story, you could have your main character find a way to resolve his or her anger. You might read books about people who have been angry after the death of a loved one. The person who says he or she has no anger is probably denying grief, and is going to be a long time getting over it. Anger is part and parcel of grief. In the space below, write three things that make you angry about your deceased loved one. Say them out loud and imagine the reply.

1. _____

_____

Reply: _____

_____

2. _____

_____

Reply: _____

_____

3. _____

_____

Reply: _____

_____

3. Set limits.

Part of your anger comes from the overwhelming and timeless dimensions of grief. It's like being put into a cage from which there is seemingly no escape. A ritual provides you with an activity that has a beginning and an end, as well as a clear purpose. It puts you in control.

This list of suggested rituals includes many found helpful by others. What works for one may not necessarily work for another. A ritual that you create yourself will be the most helpful.

- Have a schedule for watering, misting and pruning plants. Get a moisture meter and set a certain time each day for tending to your plants.
- Polish silver, brass, or copper items on certain days and at specific times.
- Wash the car on Monday, wax on Tuesday, check the tires on Wednesday, get gas and check the oil on Thursday, vacuum and dust the inside on Friday, and on Saturday go somewhere special.
- Clean a cupboard or a closet, just one, every day at the same time.
- Set aside an hour each day to work on sorting through boxes of snapshots. Search out documents, certificates, diplomas, and other memorabilia pertaining to your loved one. Using these things, along with your own written remembrances, make a book of his or her life.

- If someone in your family is having a baby, make a quilt, afghan, or a wooden toy for the baby.
- Give two or three hours a week to an organization you would like to support.
- Have a special time each day for cataloging your books. Make a card file and place the books on the shelves in order.
- Now list some ideas of your own. Rituals diffuse anger nonaggressively.

_____

_____

_____

_____

_____

Rituals come more easily if you are a bit compulsive anyway. For those who are not, it may take a few false starts to really get into it. You may, in fact, wonder if rituals will make the compulsive person more compulsive. My experience is that it lessens compulsivity. Grief is a unique state. What normally applies may have to be reconsidered when you are in grief.

Receiving Love

When someone dies, you feel rejected. You feel unloved and unloveable. Even when there's ample evidence to the contrary, you can't see it. This way of thinking is illogical and irrational, but no amount of explanation is going to change the way you feel. When someone loses a leg or an eye, these same feelings of being unloveable may occur. The beloved person was a part of you, and now he or she is inexplicably not present. You can get out of this state, and it's important that you do. Being able to receive love again is a big step in grief work. The following exercise is designed to help you receive love. I'm defining love as any gesture which might indicate that someone cares about you. This could be a warm smile, a pat on the back, a hug, or verbal expressions of love and concern. Don't analyze these gestures for sincerity; accept them unconditionally as gestures of love. That does not mean, of course, accepting any gesture that makes you feel uncomfortable. You always have a right to turn down gestures that feel wrong to you. Most likely you will find that you can receive love from some people and tend to reject it from others. Awareness of your ability to receive love will help you begin to open up to receiving love.

 Examine the "Monitoring Feelings" exercise on the next page. This is less an exercise to do here than a perspective to bring out into the world with you. As you meet people, or talk with them on the phone during the day, make mental notes about the exercise questions. When you have a chance, use the space provided to reflect on your attitudes and experiences. Do this every week until you feel the love being offered you. When you feel that, the bad feeling of unloveableness will diminish.

Monitoring Feelings

1. Choose a day this week when you are willing to receive love. Circle the day below:

   Sunday Monday Tuesday Wednesday Thursday Friday Saturday

2. On that day, be aware of all interactions, verbal and nonverbal. Ask yourself these questions:

- How willing am I to receive love? Am I open to friendly gestures, or do I withdraw into myself? _____
  _____
  _____

- How did I feel after the most recent loving gesture? Frightened? Glad? What?
  _____
  _____
  _____

3. At the end of the day, review and notice the conditions of each interaction.

- With whom was it OK to be loved? (*i.e.*, the girl on the playground, the man in the drugstore, the paper boy, and so forth). _____
  _____
  _____

- When it wasn't OK, what was I afraid of? Afraid to be vulnerable? Afraid something would be expected of me? Afraid of having to return gestures of love? _____
  _____
  _____

- Were any gestures legitimately unsafe or inappropriate? _____
  _____
  _____

- How many times do I reject love? One to three times a day? Five times?
  _____
  _____
  _____

- Is there anything I can do about it? _____
  _____
  _____

Letting Go of Guilt

Even the kindest and best-intentioned person will feel guilt after someone dies. Grief triggers the brain to go over and over everything that was ever said and done, looking for causes for the death. No one gets through life without having moments of impatience. No one makes it to the end without saying a cross word. Most of us say a good many cross words. Every word becomes magnified into a monstrous deed that caused the beloved person sadness. You remember with horror the day you asked a neighbor to sit with your dying husband so you could escape to the mall for an hour. "How could I have been so selfish," you say. "He must have thought I hated taking care of him." Tossing sleeplessly you process all of these things, and the sickening guilt grows.

Under normal circumstances you are probably able to recognize your human condition, accept your mistakes, and avoid magnifying those things that are not mistakes. When grief comes, all that reasonable thinking goes out the window. Even though your husband died of cancer, you begin to think, "He willed himself to die. Life with me was unbearable and he couldn't escape."

Some guilt in life is necessary, a friendly nudge to set you on the right path. The guilt that comes with grief can make you sick. It works like an insidious poison. The only cure is to be able to sort out the little guilt that helps you grow and become a better person from the big, exaggerated, illogical guilt that makes you sick. There is a pathway through this maze. It is a hard and painful path, but if you stay with it to the end, you will be rewarded.

The Guilt Maze

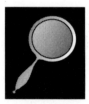

In the exercise that follows you will see plenty of blank space. This is your space to fill with the words, actions, and thoughts feeding your guilt. You will create a maze, following your own design. Eventually, you will find your way out of this maze. Follow the four steps below, taking as much time as you need.

1. *Start* by writing down every word, every action, and every thought that's making you feel guilty. Leave nothing out. Put things in any order you like. This will hurt, and you will cry, but the tears are healing tears. Get a big box of tissue and get started.

2. *Wander* through your guilt maze. Can you cross out anything? Are there some words, thoughts, actions that every normal person would likely do in similar circumstances? If you think you can cross something out, say to yourself, "I can let that go. That is normal behavior. No one would take lasting offense at that." Go over and over it again until you feel comfortable with what you have done.

3. Now go over your maze and circle those words, thoughts, and actions from which you can learn something. These will be things that are deeply hurtful, and the guilt may be very strong. Husbands and wives, fathers and sons, mothers and daughters — in every relationship people hurt each other at times. It's OK to feel bad about those things because you can learn from them. It is by making mistakes that people build strong relationships. If no one ever felt bad about doing hurtful things to another, there would be no way to create a lasting, loving relationship.

When Hilda did the guilt maze exercise a few months after her husband died at home, she found that most of the guilt she had was unjustified. She had been cross at times when she was tired. Once she didn't get up in the night when her husband called; she was exhausted to the point of being nonfunctional. Another time she said she was going shopping for an hour and stayed out three hours. The thought of going back home to the sounds and sights and smells of illness was more than she could handle. By staying away three hours, she was able to pull herself together; she gathered strength to handle a job that only she could do. As Hilda wrote about these things, she knew Bob had understood her need and was not hurt.

Then she remembered the terrible night when she had been up all night with Bob. He was demanding water, urinal, back rub, something every 15 minutes. When he dropped the full urinal on the floor, something in Hilda snapped. "I wish this would be over with," she mumbled. Bob heard. The anguished look in Bob's eyes haunted Hilda's waking thoughts and her dreams. Writing about this episode elicited a burst of sobs. Hilda cried wildly until she was worn out. She realized then that she could be hurtful under stress. She recognized that most people would be this way. But she also knew that she didn't want it to happen again, and she wished she could apologize to Bob.

Now this is the important thing: even though your loved one is dead, you still have the relationship. If you still have a relationship, then you can still improve it. Think about the following questions, reflecting on your feelings and experiences.

- How do you improve a relationship after you have done something hurtful?
- How do you seek forgiveness from the person you have wronged?
- How do you forgive the person who has wronged you?
- How do you forgive yourself?
- What will you be doing differently now, not only in this relationship, but in other relationships as well?

4. *Finish* the maze by taking action to correct behaviors which have been destructive in any relationship. The action steps Hilda remembered and resolved to repeat are these:

- I will write a letter to Bob.
- I will say how I felt, and I will tell him that I'm sorry I hurt him. I will tell him how much I love him and miss him.
- I will make peace with myself through prayer and meditation.
- I will begin to forgive myself for human frailty, and I will be more observant of how other people are feeling before I speak.

Hilda also wrote a statement of commitment based on her experience: "When I am under stress, I will step away from the situation long enough to become calm. I will not speak until I am in control."

Perhaps some lists of words and actions will help you to formulate your own statement of commitment.

Feelings

angry	sad	lonely	desperate
hopeless	helpless	frustrated	anguished
forsaken	forgotten	confused	guilty
abused	vindictive	frightened	dumped on

Actions

assertively confront	take time out
write in my journal	write to someone
clean house	apologize
ask for an apology	express appreciation
ask forgiveness	give forgiveness
talk with someone who can be objective	go on with my life

Statement of Commitment

When I feel_____I will do/say/write_____,
and_____, and allow myself to remember_____
_____.

Now list concrete steps you can take to carry out this commitment.

1. I will do _____
2. I will say _____
3. I will make _____
4. I will give up _____
5. I will begin _____

You are not going to do all of these things in a week, or maybe not in a month. For one thing, you won't have the energy. For another, it would be too painful to do too much of this all at once. It's going to take up to a year or more to let go of anger and guilt and be able to receive and give love. Take your time. Work on one step at a time.

Getting Help

Normal grief is not a pathological condition. It can turn into an illness if you don't allow yourself to experience it fully and work it through. Denying it won't make it go away. It'll be there waiting for you, ready to pop up bigger and more painful than ever. Probably this would happen when you are under stress or the next time you lose someone you love. Delayed grief is very hard to handle. Don't cover it up with busyness. Your business right now is to see it through.

If grief turns into clinical depression, you will need professional help. Symptoms of depression include: major change in appetite, unusual weight loss or gain, constant crying, constipation, inability to do daily tasks or to socialize, disinterest in appearance. If these symptoms persist for more than a month, it would be well to seek help. Thoughts of suicide mean you need help right now. Suicide is a thoughtless and cruel act. It hurts everyone you love for the rest of their lives, and it doesn't solve anything. If you have such thoughts, please call your doctor *now*, even if it's Sunday or his golf day, or it's the middle of the night. Ask for a referral to a grief counselor.

Nearly every hospital has a hospice. The bereavement counselor there can direct you to the kind of help you need. Using the services of a bereavement counselor can be good prevention, too. By having someone guide you through grief, you can protect yourself from major depression.

Every death is different. Every survivor is unique. Circumstances of the death make a difference in how grief is experienced. The suggestions in this book are for the kind of grief most commonly experienced. When there have been abusive relationships or uncommonly invasive procedures done to the dying person, grief may take on a different character. If you feel in need of help, then you should get it. Your doctor or someone from your church may be able to help you. There are also many books to read, and for some that is therapeutic. A list of grief books are included in the References section at the end of this chapter.

Your life will go on. You determine what kind of life that will be. Resolve now to make decisions that will give you control until the end. Make decisions now that will make it easier for you to bear the final illness of a loved one. You are the one who has to do it. You are the one who can choose to continue living, loving, and growing.

Like Alice, you have been through the looking glass into your own Wonderland. You may not have met a Mad hatter, but I hope you have come face-to-face with a few of your own fearful creatures (and met wonderful ones, too). Alice was different when she came back from her Wonderland. Her experiences changed her. Both sides of the looking glass had come to seem a wondrous world.

If you have leafed through this book, ideas may have struck that you'd like to explore further. If you have read each chapter thoroughly and worked through the self-reflection exercises, you have already progressed far in your explorations. Perhaps you have found new strengths in yourself, and recognized old ones. Perhaps you have found new uses for these strengths. At least, I hope you have come to see how much control and power you have over your own world.

Let this book serve you as your resource now. Use its guidelines on health and communication and other practical matters as you need them. Use the resources you've identified for yourself within these pages, as well. Above all, remember the people and beliefs you have identified as your supporting living system. If people want to help and love you, let them do so. If your beliefs are a solace and a guide, follow them.

My own adventure through the looking glassand into the writing of this book, has been one of growing wonder, a sense of connectedness with you, and with people everywhere. I have enjoyed this and profited greatly. I hope you have, too.

References

Arnold, J.H., and P. Buschman Gemma (1983) *A Child Dies: A Portrait of Family Grief.* Rockville, MD: Aspen Systems Corporation.

Birkedahl, N. (1985) *Grief...A Pathway to Personal Growth and Self-Awareness.* Grand Junction, CO: Hilltop Rehabilitation Hospital Hospice.

Committee for the Study of Health Consequences of the Stress of Bereavement/Institute of Medicine (1984) *Bereavement: Reactions, Consequences, and Care.* Edited by M. Osterweis, F. Solomon, and M. Green. Washington, D.C.: National Academy Press.

Kubler-Ross, E. (1969) *On Death and Dying.* New York: Macmillan Publishing Co., Inc.

Kubler-Ross, E. (1974) *Question and Answers on Death and Dying.* New York: Macmillan Publishing Co., Inc.

Nouwen, H.J.M. (1980) *In Memoriam.* Notre Dame, IN: Ave Maria Press.

Rando, T.A. (1984) *Grief, Dying, and Death.* Champaign, IL: Research Press Co.

Roach, N. (1974) *The Last Day of April.* American Cancer Society.

Schoenberg, B., A.C. Carr, D. Peretz, and A.H. Kuscher (1970) *Loss and Grief.* New York: Columbia University Press.

Appendix

Contacts and Resources for Answering Your Questions

This list of resources contains names, addresses, and phone numbers of places you can contact for information and support. Most are tailored to the needs of the elderly, but some offer broad-based services to people who share a specific interest. Don't hesitate to call or write, even if you're not sure they can help with a particular concern. If they can't help, they'll be able to refer you to another person or agency who can give you what you need. Think of this quest for information as an adventure, a journey down a path that may lead you to something unexpected and wonderful.

Remember that there are other resources close at hand, such as newspapers, phone-books, and libraries. Many of the organizations listed below have local chapters, and there just might be one in your city. You are not alone, your problems and concerns are most likely shared by some other people. You might find yourself giving solace and help as well as receiving it.

Advocacy Groups

Coalition of Advocates for Rights of Infirm Elderly (CARIE)
1315 Walnut St., Suite 900
Philadelphia, PA 19107
215-545-5728
(Telephone referral service for older people who are disabled or infirm.)

The Hastings Center
360 Broadway
Hastings-on-Hudson
New York, NY 10706
914-762-8500
(Issues of aging: moral issues of medical technology, dying, national health care, and long-term care.)

Arts

National Center on Arts and Aging
c/o National Council on Aging
600 Maryland Ave. SW
Washington, D.C. 20024
202-479-1200, Ext. 387 or 259
(Heads a national campaign to increase involvement of senior citizens in the arts.)

Children and Family of Aging Parents

Children of Aging Parents
2761 Trenton Rd.
Levittown, PA 19056
215-547-1070
(Provides information on housing and caregiving for children and families of seniors. Send self-addressed, stamped envelope for information.)

Communications Services

Lifeline Systems
1-800-451-0525
in Alaska, Hawaii, and Massachusetts: 617-923-4141
(Information on Lifeline Systems, an emergency telephone system for senior citizens.)

Tele-Consumer Hotline
1-800-332-1124
in Washington, D.C.: 202-483-4100
(Answers questions on your telephone service and equipment and tells you where to go to find further assistance, ways to cut costs, and solutions to billing problems.)

Concerned Caregivers

American College of Health Care Administration (ACHCA)
325 S. Patrick St.
Alexandria, VA 22314
703-549-5822
(Primarily concerned with nursing home administration.)

American Geriatric Society
770 Lexington Ave., Suite 400
New York, NY 10001
212-242-0214
(An association of physicians specializing in medical treatment of older people.)

American Hospital Association
840 North Lake Shore Dr.
Chicago, IL 60611
312-280-6000
(Provides information on health care for seniors, research and education on health care administration, and more.)

American Medical Association
535 N. Dearborn St.
Chicago, IL 60610
(Advocates strict enforcement of laws protecting elderly.)

American Society for Geriatric Dentistry
1121 West Michigan St.
Indianapolis, IN 46202
317-264-8845
(Educates dental professionals on the needs of senior patients and offers publications.)

National Hospice Organization
1901 North Fort Myer Dr., Suite 307
Arlington, VA 22209
703-243-5900
(Encourages training of hospice care personnel and has pamphlets.)

Consumer Issues

Better Business Bureaus
1515 Wilson Blvd.
Arlington, VA 33309
703-276-0100
(Consumer protection offering pamphlets on: funerals, hearing aids, land scams, and more.)

Consumer Information Center
P.O. Box 100
Pueblo, CO 81002
(Education and information office of the federal government. Provides free or low-cost pamphlets on a wide variety of topics including housing, drugs and food safety, home safety, wise buying practices, home repair, and more.)

Food and Drug Administration
5600 Fishers Ln.
Rockville, MD 20856
301-443-3170
(This federal agency provides extensive information on food, drugs, and cosmetics.)

United Seniors Consumer Cooperative
1334 G St. NW, Suite 500
Washington D.C. 20005
202-393-6222
(Nonprofit organization that offers extensive health care information and low-cost services to older members nationwide. Extensive computer base tells you the best doctors, dentists, or medical specialists in your area. Analyzes medi-gap insurance plans available in your state and offers a special service to remind you of annual physical or dates for medical tests.)

Education

Arthritis Service Network
Arthritis Foundation
1314 Spring St. NW
Atlanta, GA 30309
404-351-0454
(A health-education network offering health programs on self-help and exercise nation-wide. Call or write for pamphlets.)

Catholic Charities
1319 F St. NW, 4th Floor
Washington D.C. 20004
202-398-1022
(Sponsors educational workshops and leadership-training institutes. Provides speakers on Medicare and other subjects. Distributes films, reports, and publications.)

Elderhostel
80 Boylston St., Suite 400
Boston, MA 02116
(Provides a catalog of international schools and universities cooperating in its program of education for seniors, including living arrangements on campuses.)

National Library Service for the Blind
1-800-336-4797
Alaska, Hawaii, Virginia, Washington D.C.: collect 703-522-2590
(Operated by the Library of Congress.)
Call for information about reading materials and help with research.

Finance

Federal Deposit Insurance Corporation
1-800-424-5488
in Washington D.C.: 202-389-4473
(Information on Truth in Lending Law, banking laws, and assistance with banking complaints.)

Federal Reserve System
Board of Governors
Washington D.C. 20551
202-452-4000
(Information on banking and credit protection.)

Institute of Certified Financial Planners
9725 East Hamden Ave.
Denver, CO 80231
303-751-7600
(Referrals to qualified financial planners and a free pamphlet on guidelines for selecting a financial planner.)

National Foundation for Consumer Credit
8701 Georgia Ave., Suite 507
Silver Spring, MD 20910
1-800-589-5600
(Will give you the name and address of your state Consumer Credit Counseling Services.
Also information on credit use.)

Funeral

Continental Association of Funeral and Memorial Societies
2001 S St. NW, Suite 530
Washington D.C. 20009
(Information on how to plan and carry out simple memorial and funeral services.)

Health

Alzheimer's Disease and Related Disorders Association
1-800-621-0379
in Illinois: 1-800-572-6037
(Information on Alzheimer's Disease.)

American Council of the Blind
1-800-424-8666
(Information on causes and treatment of blindness.)

American Heart Association
7320 Greenville Ave.
Dallas, TX 75231
214-750-5397
(Publications on heart disease. Supports research on heart attack, stroke, and other heart
and blood vessel disease.)

American Kidney Fund
1-800-638-8299
in Maryland: 1-800-492-8361
in Washington D.C.: 1-301-986-1444
(Information on kidney disease.)

American Osteopathic Association
142 E. Ontario St.
Chicago, IL 60611
312-208-5800
(General information about osteopathic medicine and referral sources to practitioners.)

Arthritis Foundation
3400 Peachtree Rd., NE, Room 1101
Atlanta, GA 30326
404-351-0454
(Arthritis research: offers publications, and operates Arthritis Service Network.)

BYU Senior Help Line
Brigham Young University
F-274 Harris Fine Arts Center
Provo, UT 84602
1-800-328-7576
(Informative messages on more than 100 topics of interest to older adults and caregivers. Free throughout the United States, Canada, and Puerto Rico. Written copies of messages, as well as braille directories, are available at no charge. Call for list of topics.)

Cancer Information Service
1-800-4-CANCER
in Washington D.C.: 202-636-5700
(Information on all forms of cancer, and answers to questions about problems related to cancer.)

Continence Restored, Inc.
785 Park Ave.
New York, NY 10021
(Associated with Help for Incontinent People. Sponsors support groups nationwide for people suffering from urinary incontinence. Send self-addressed, stamped legal-size envelope for information.)

Dial-a-Hearing Screening Test
1-800-222-EARS
in Pennsylvania: 215-565-6114
(Information on hearing problems.)

Help for Incontinent People
P.O. Box 544
Union, SC 29379
(Publishes a quarterly newsletter for $5 a year, and a Resource Guide of Continence Aids and Services for $3.)

High Blood Pressure Information Center
120-80 National Institutes of Health
Bethesda, MD 20882
301-496-1809
(Information on detection, diagnosis, and treatment of high blood pressure.)

Lung Line
1-800-222-LUNG
(Information on lung disease.)

Medic Alert Foundation
1-800-344-3226
California: 1-800-468-1020
in Alaska, Hawaii: 209-668-3333
(Information about an identification bracelet listing health condition, medications, allergies, and doctor's numbers. Helps medical personnel provide care in an emergency.)

National Health Information Center
P.O. Box 1133
Washington D.C. 20013
703-522-2590
(Provides printed information and referrals.)

National Institute of Neurological and Communicative Disorders and Stroke
Building 31, Room 8A06
Bethesda, MD 20892
301-496-5751 or 496-5924
(Research on communicative and neurological disorders and stroke. Provides grants to institutions and individuals in related fields. Send for publications.)

National Institute on Drug Abuse
5600 Fishers Ln., Room 10A43
Rockville, MD 20857
(Information on drug abuse, including accidental misuse of prescription drugs by older people.)

Nutribionics
Box 959
Washington, UT 84780
1-800-852-8280
in Utah: 801-673-8885
(Information on the science of body tissue regeneration.)

Housing

American Association of Homes for the Aging (AAHA)
1129 20th St. NW, Suite 400
Washington D.C. 20036
202-783-2242
(Information about residential facilities for older people.)

B'nai B'rith International
1640 Rhode Island Ave. NW
Washington, D.C. 20036
202-857-6600
(Involved in retirement planning and senior housing programs. Also provides consumer guidance for seniors and offers publications.)

Shared Housing Resource Center
6344 Greene St.
Philadelphia, PA 19144
(Information and publications on shared housing.)

Insurance

Federal Crime Insurance Hotline
1-800-638-8780
in Alaska, Hawaii, Maryland, call collect: 0-301-652-2637
(Eligibility for federally subsidized crime insurance in participating states. Helps individuals who are denied burglary and robbery insurance.)

Health Care Financing Administration
Department of Health and Human Services
Baltimore, MD 21207
301-966-3000
(Excellent publications on Medicare.)

Legal

Legal Counsel for the Elderly
c/o AARP
1909 K St. NW
Washington D.C. 20049
202-234-0970
(Self-help legal information for older people.)

National Association of State Units of Aging
600 Maryland Ave. SW, Suite 208, West Wing
Washington D.C. 20024
202-484-7182
(Provides information on current legislative and regulatory issues and policies affecting state aging programs. Send for publications.)

Social Security, Pensions, Federal Taxes, Welfare

IRS Taxpayer Assistance
1-800-424-1040
(Information on problems and questions about taxes.)

Pension Rights Center
1701 K St. NW
Washington D.C. 20006
(Publications about pension rights.)

Save Our Security (SOS)
Coalition to Protect Social Security
1201 16th St. NW, Suite 222
Washington D.C. 20036
(Lobbies for legislative measures which will safeguard social security system.)

Social Security Hotline
1-800-662-1111
(Information on Social Security benefits and federal income taxes.)

U.S. Department of Labor
Pension and Welfare Benefit Programs
Office of Communications, Room N4662
200 Constitution Ave. NW
Washington D.C. 20210
(Information about the rights of senior citizens under federal private-pension laws.)

Special Interest Groups for Seniors

Organization of Chinese Americans
2025 Eye St. NW, Suite 926
Washington D.C. 20006
(Promotes equal opportunity for Chinese Americans. Send for publications, including *The Elderly Chinese: A Forgotten Minority*.)

National Association for Hispanic Elderly
(Asociacion Nacional Pro Personas Mayores)
1730 West Olympic Blvd., Suite 401
Los Angeles, CA 90015
213-487-1922
(Assists Hispanic seniors. Offers technical assistance and training for older workers. Ask for publications.)

National Caucus and Center on Black Aged
1424 K St. NW, Suite 500
Washington D.C. 20005
202-637-8400
(Information on employment, housing, and improvement of social services. Technical assistance and training to minority sponsors for the elderly. Transportation and development of the Black Voluntary Networks.)

National Pacific/Asian Resource Center on Aging
811 First Ave.
Colman Building, Suite 210
Seattle, WA 98104
206-622-5124
(Seeks to improve health services for the Pacific-Asian community. Send for publications.)

National Rehabilitation Information Center
1-800-34NARIC
(Information about products to make life easier for disabled persons.)

National Urban League
500 East 62nd St.
New York, NY 10021
212-310-9000
(Seeks to eliminate racial discrimination. Sponsors a health promotion project and provides assistance to local groups. Send for publications.)

Veterans Administration
1-800-622-4134
(Information to veterans and their dependents on benefits for education, health care, disability, and retirement.)

Travel

American Society of Travel Agents, Inc.
4400 MacArthur Blvd. NW
Washington D.C. 20007
202-965-7520
(Free literature, such as: *The United States Welcomes Handicapped Visitors.*)

Volunteer Programs

Service Corps of Retired Executives
1129 Twentieth St. NW, Suite 410
Washington D.C. 20036
(Matches the experience of retired business people with small businesses needing help, on a volunteer basis.)

Volunteer Hotlines
1-800-424-8580
in Alaska and Hawaii: 1-800-424-9704
(Information on the Peace Corps and VISTA volunteers. For specific information on Older American Volunteer programs, such as Foster Grandparents, Senior Companions, and Retired Senior Volunteer programs, call 1-800-424-8867; Washington D.C.: 202-634-9355.)

American Association of Retired Persons (AARP)
1909 K St. NW
Washington D.C. 20049
202-434-2277
(Publications, informative brochures about health, travel, social security, medicare and more. Lobbies for age-related issues.)

Other New Harbinger Self-Help Titles

Older & Wiser: A Workbook for Coping With Aging, $12.95

Prisoners of Belief: Exposing & Changing Beliefs that Control Your Life, $10.95

Be Sick Well: A Healthy Approach to Chronic Illness, $11.95

Men & Grief: A Guide for Men Surviving the Death of a Loved One, $11.95

When the Bough Breaks: A Helping Guide for Parents of Sexually Abused Childern, $11.95

Love Addiction: A Guide to Emotional Independence, $11.95

When Once Is Not Enough: Help for Obsessive Compulsives, $11.95

The New Three Minute Meditator, $9.95

Getting to Sleep, $10.95

The Relaxation & Stress Reduction Workbook, 3rd Edition, $13.95

Leader's Guide to the Relaxation & Stress Reduction Workbook, $19.95

Beyond Grief: A Guide for Recovering from the Death of a Loved One, $10.95

Thoughts & Feelings: The Art of Cognitive Stress Intervention, $13.95

Messages: The Communication Skills Book, $12.95

The Divorce Book, $11.95

Hypnosis for Change: A Manual of Proven Techniques, 2nd Edition, $12.95

The Deadly Diet: Recovering from Anorexia & Bulimia, $11.95

Self-Esteem, $12.95

Acquiring Courage: An Audio Cassette for the Rapid Treatment of Phobias, $14.95

The Better Way to Drink, $11.95

Chronic Pain Control Workbook, $13.95

Rekindling Desire: Bringing Your Sexual Relationship Back to Life, $12.95

Life Without Fear: Anxiety and Its Cure, $10.95

Visualization for Change, $12.95

Guideposts to Meaning: Discovering What Really Matters, $11.95

Controlling Stagefright, $11.95

Videotape: Clinical Hypnosis for Stress & Anxiety Reduction, $24.95

Starting Out Right: Essential Parenting Skills for Your Child's First Years, $12.95

Big Kids: A Parent's Guide to Weight Control for Children, $11.95

Personal Peace: Transcending Your Interpersonal Limits, $11.95

My Parent's Keeper: Adult Children of the Emotionally Disturbed, $11.95

When Anger Hurts, $12.95

Free of the Shadows: Recovering from Sexual Violence, $12.95

Resolving Conflict With Others and Within Yourself, $12.95

Liftime Weight Control, $11.95

The Anxiety & Phobia Workbook, $13.95

Love and Renewal: A Couple's Guide to Commitment, $12.95

The Habit Control Workbook, $12.95

Send a check for the titles you want, plus $2.00 for shipping and handling, to:

New Harbinger Publications, Inc.
5674 Shattuck Avenue
Oakland, CA 94609

Or write for a free catalog of all our quality self-help publications. For orders over $20 call 1-800-748-6273. Have your Visa or Mastercard number ready.